Enio Figueira Junior

Mouth breathing as a consequence of respiratory sensitivity

Enio Figueira Junior

Mouth breathing as a consequence of respiratory sensitivity

House dust mites as a cause of respiratory and skin allergies

ScienciaScripts

Imprint

Cover image: www.ingimage.com

This book is a translation from the original published under ISBN 978-613-9-72078-1.

Publisher:
Sciencia Scripts
is a trademark of
Dodo Books Indian Ocean Ltd. and OmniScriptum S.R.L publishing group

120 High Road, East Finchley, London, N2 9ED, United Kingdom
Str. Armeneasca 28/1, office 1, Chisinau MD-2012, Republic of Moldova, Europe
Printed at: see last page
ISBN: 978-620-7-94092-9

DEDICATORY

I offer this work first of all to God, for his light in the face of so many obstacles that have come my way;

I would also like to thank my wife Ana Célia for understanding my absence at times. My love has not diminished, it has increased.

To Professor Gilberto Salles de Gazêta for his support and guidance in the development of this work.

To Dr Oscarina da Silva Ezequiel for her help in applying and interpreting the allergens.

To our patients, for the true patience they had to have because of the various tests that had to be carried out during the course of the work.

SUMMARY

According to the literature, mouth breathing originates from an obstruction of the nasal passages and early diagnosis of this condition aims to minimise and even eliminate the skeletal and organic alterations that result. The ratio of mouth breathers as a result of respiratory hypersensitivity caused by dust mites has been shown to be high, especially in the younger age groups, during periods of bone development, giving rise to Mouth Breathing (MB).

Out of a total of 40 people assessed, regardless of age, race, sex, occupation and domicile, coming from the most diverse places, from private practices to hospitals in the Unified Health System, an initial selection was made based on clinical characteristics, resulting in a total of 32 patients. This was followed by a single protocol for all the patients: clinical examination, anamnesis, specific radiographic tests, examination of salivary characteristics and immediate reading skin tests to detect and characterise the allergic source.

Mites were present as stimulants of allergic conditions in almost all age groups in the sample examined, and the *Dermatophagoides pteronyssinus* mite stood out as the most constant species.

CONTENTS

CHAPTER 1

INTRODUCTION

Breathing is an innate and reflex function that is characterised by its rhythmic realisation, an uninterrupted succession of ventilatory cycles. The inhaled air needs to be filtered to prevent impurities from entering through the nostrils, and by heating and humidifying it, to make it ideal for travelling all the way to the lungs. The cilia located in the nostrils are responsible for blocking impurities, preventing them from reaching the lungs so that the body can make the most of them. In the normal sequence, air enters through the nose, goes to the pharynx, then to the larynx, trachea and bronchi, finally reaching the pulmonary alveoli, allowing mainly for the intake or supply of the necessary O_2 , and the elimination of CO_2 ; thus promoting ventilation control. This is called the Ventilatory Cycle or Respiratory Cycle, where each cycle comprises an inspiration and an expiration. This Respiratory Cycle leads to the development of the body's structures, from birth onwards, by a corresponding force of distension x pulmonary tension; this force promotes bone modelling and a growth stimulus, as a result of essential muscular actions (MARCHESAN, 1998; RIOS, 1996).

Mouth breathing is the act of an individual breathing more frequently through the oral cavity because the nasal cavity and adjacent organic structures are causing alterations in normal respiratory function. A mouth breather, by definition, is an individual who has deviated from the normal nasal breathing pattern and consequently has mixed breathing. Mouth-only breathing is considered very rare (QUELUZ & GIMENEZ, 2000; RIOS, 1996).

Mouth breathing (MB) arises from obstruction of the upper airways due to various causes, including abscesses and tumours, nasal polyps, deviated septum and incorrect posture, as well as allergic rhinitis. This change in the respiratory mechanism leads to adaptive changes in the dental arches and surrounding tissues (QUELUZ & GIMENEZ, 2000; FERREIRA, 1998; MOCELLIN, 1994). Despite the multifactorial causes, MARCHESAN (1998) draws attention to the high frequency of RB with respiratory allergies (ARNOLT et al, 1991). However, the intrinsic relationship between patients with type I hypersensitivity reactions, resulting in RB and subsequent alterations in the function of organs and tissues as a whole, is rarely found in the literature. On the contrary, several studies, previously and separately published, are restricted to specific areas of interest without, however, qualifying the etiology of MB. Evaluations of mouth breathing in relation to respiratory allergies have taken morphofunctional alterations into account (QUELUZ & GIMENEZ, 2000; CINTRA et al, 2000; OLIVEIRA et al, 1998; RIZZO, 1998; SABRA & MARTINS, 1997; MORENO et al, 1995).

Prevalent mouth breathing tends to lead to bone alterations, so that the prematurity of the process influences the level and quantity of the alterations, which occur from an early age, during the child's first years of growth. Early diagnosis is therefore aimed at achieving correct bone modelling. This early diagnosis increases the possibility of preventative activities; otherwise, the condition gradually worsens (CINTRA et al, 2000; LUSVARGHI, 1999; RIOS, 1996; ARAGÃO, 1986). The clinical picture presented by mouth breathing calls for multi-professional action since it is not possible to establish where one action begins and, at the end of it, another begins, and so on and so forth. In view of this, each professional in their specific area is responsible for part of the importance of their examination for a final diagnosis, which is multidisciplinary. An otorhinolaryngologist's examination aims to correct the difficulty in normal nasal breathing by finding its cause, in association with an allergist when necessary. However, once this direct cause has been removed, the patient still has the habit of breathing through the mouth and needs respiratory re-education. In this respiratory re-education, which is the main point of the treatment, a change in the current way of breathing must really be achieved by a speech therapist. Any orthodontic correction made before respiratory re-education runs the risk of treatment relapse, as the habit is maintained by the individual (LUSVARGHI, 1999; DI FRANCESCO, 1999; FERREIRA, 1998).

This difficulty in breathing by normal means leads the body to promote skeletal changes as an adaptation to a new situation, leading to other relevant changes (CINTRA et al., 2000; RIZZO, 1998; SABRA & MARTINS, 1997).

Currently, the climatic changes that the world has been going through, due to absurdly high levels of air pollution, which have reached regions that were previously free of them, have led to the increase and emergence of various pathologies, including those associated with certain parasites and insects, which until then had been restricted to living in certain areas (MORENO et al., 1995). The organism, in turn, needs to adapt to these new situations. We are trying to understand which changes are responsible for changes in immunological responses to allergens. House dust, despite its name, does not originate purely in the home, but from particles suspended in the atmosphere in anthropogenic ecosystems. Mites and some parasites, found in different anthropogenic environments, find in this household dust a real substrate for their development where, associated with dust of the most diverse origins, they initiate the so-called allergic processes in humans (RIZZO.1998; FACCINI et aL, 1991), especially those that produce alterations in respiratory physiology.

Wide access to the places where dust mites thrive, due to their characteristics, sensitises people who are already predisposed to developing respiratory problems.

Most of the research carried out to diagnose patients with type I hypersensitivity reactions looks for the cause, the main origin of which is dust mites, leading to the development of allergic rhinitis and, in an exacerbated process, asthma, without there being any interrelationship between the two (DI FRANCESCO,1999; AALBERSE.1998SABRA & MARTINS, 1997; GELLER,

1996; MORENO et al, 1995; VOORHORST et al, 1969 Apud MORENO et al, 1995; KONISHI & UEHARA, 1994; ANDRADE etaL, 1991).

In the increase observed in the prevalence of asthma in the world between 1960 and 1995, in addition to other factors, the increase in exposure to allergens is considered to be of great importance.

CHAPTER 2

OBJECTIVE

The aim of this study was to observe the correlation between mouth breathing (MB) and allergic reactions caused by dust mites by analysing the various aetiological factors that limit this functional alteration.

CHAPTER 3

LITERATURE REVIEW

The association of Household Ecosystem Mites (HEE) with respiratory and cutaneous allergic diseases is indisputable (EZEQUIEL.2000). The families Pyroglyphidae, Glycyphagidae, Acaridae and Cheyletidae stand out (MAUNSELL et aL, 1968; SUMMERS & PRICE, 1970; COHEN, 1980; FELDMAN-MUHSAM et aL, 1985; GALVÃO & GUITTON, 1986; FAIN et aL, 1990; NASPITZ et aL, 1990; GOMES, 1991; BERND etaL, 1994; COLOFF, 1998; GELLER, 1999).

Allergy to house dust caused by mites of the genus *Dermatophagoides spp.* has been proven for some time; they can cause, on their own, or aggravate respiratory allergy (GALVÃO & GUITTON, 1986; FAIN et al, 1990; BERND et al, 1994; GELLER, 1996; GELLER, 1999).

This literature review looked at the various aspects involved in mouth breathing, its main causes, its relationship with certain allergens and its consequences. The specific action of mites and their consequences was assessed due to the worldwide distribution of this arthropod (MORENO et aL,1995).

Respiratory diseases are among the most frequent health problems today, and both asthma and allergic rhinitis affect a large percentage of children and adults. The environment is of great importance as it has been acting on the respiratory tract as a potential risk factor for the development of these diseases (RIZZO,1998).

HERMANN et al (2013) confirmed the occurrence of these alterations in the maxillo-mandibular complex in children and emphasised the importance of dentists working to prevent caries and periodontal disease, pathologies that are commonly associated with mouth breathers.

HERMANN et al (2013) also state that the submission of these patients to allergic skin tests (prick-test) allows the adoption of measures to reduce these allergens that cause mouth breathing

3.1 - The relationship between mouth breathing and allergies and/or rhinitis.

The importance of studying pathologies other than allergic rhinitis, such as rhinoconjunctivitis and sinusitis, lies in the fact that house dust mites are capable of compromising individuals on a large scale, as prevalent aetiological factors. In addition to these pathologies themselves, there are complications such as secondary bacterial infections, changes in phonation, orthodontic functional anatomical compromises and changes in the quality of sleep and learning, leading to a loss of quality of life (FRANKLAND & EL-HEFNY, 1971; CUTHBERT et aL, 1979; GELLER, 1990, NEGREIROS & ESPÍNOLA, 1995; GELLER et aL, 1995; PHILIP & NACLERIO, 1996; FRIEDLAENDER, 1996; PASSÀLI & MÕSGES, 1999).

According to MARCHESAN (1998), patients who breathe more through their mouths are among those with a tendency for the face to grow more vertically, making this alteration more pronounced in these individuals; while, on the other hand, however little the nasal cavities are used in the breathing process, they bring great benefits to the normal development of the face, even in patients with allergies.

Mouth Breathing, according to DI FRANCESCO (1999), is a pathological condition associated with multiple factors, which lead to the need for a multidisciplinary approach and, once the reason for the nasal obstruction is known, there can be a better discussion of behaviour between the various professionals. LUSVARGHI (1999) emphasises that the most common cause of RB is airway obstruction, usually caused by allergic problems; these patients generally have symptoms such as nasal congestion, sneezing and rhinorrhoea.

3.2 - Rhinitis vs. allergens.

Sensitisers or allergens are, according to RIZZO (1998), *"foreign proteins or chemical substances of small molecular weight capable of inducing a Th2-type immune response and IgE-class antibodies".*

A Th2-type immune response means that there has been activation of the T-helper 2 lymphocyte. Triggers are agents that can induce an increase in airway resistance within approximately 20 minutes of exposure, without a subsequent inflammatory response. Exposure to endotoxins with these characteristics is an important determinant of symptoms among asthmatic and allergic patients (RIZZO, 1998).

Knowledge about the sources of allergens, their aerodynamic characteristics and the distribution of particle sizes are essential, since their differences weigh heavily on the study models to be developed due to their own characteristics. The great neurovegetative innervation through the nerve fibres present in the nasal mucosa leads to a particular predisposition of this mucosa to allergic shock, since its own vascular richness contributes to triggering the whole process, even extending to the paranasal cavities (CONSENSO BRASILEIRO, 1998; RIBEIRO & IRULEGUI, 1991a,b; OPAS,1989).

Allergic Rhinitis is *"a functional alteration that takes place in the nasal mucosa due to an immuno-allergic mechanism"* (OSTOLAZA.1993), and is not seen as a disease that is simply common, without major consequences, when considering its prevalence, complications and economic impact (SHELDON & SPECTOR, 1997; EZEQUIEL.2000).

Allergic Rhinitis is the result of an immediate type I hypersensitivity reaction, mediated by IgE, against inhaled allergens or food (TSUJI, 1997). It is the main cause of nasal obstruction, affecting around 15% to 20% of children and adolescents, out of a world population affected by around 10% (CINTRA et al., 2000). In the United States, it affects approximately 20% of the population and several studies have pointed out that its incidence in asthmatic adults may be around 58%, and an association has been observed between allergic rhinitis and clinical conditions such as asthma, sinusitis, otitis media, nasal polyposis, respiratory infections and dental malocclusions (SHELDON &

SPECTOR, 1997).

The typical picture of allergic rhinitis can be listed as follows: rhinorrhoea and nasal obstruction, with sternutatory crises, which can also be associated with conjunctivitis. When rhinorrhoea sets in, the child is susceptible to numerous infections of the ear, sinuses or lungs, and the adult is less able to perform activities that require greater effort (BERNARD, 1986; GELLER, 1990; PASSÀLI & MÕSGES, 1999).

These conditions, as a result of exposure to dust mites and their allergens, are characterised as generally low-grade, chronic exposure, occurring predominantly at night during sleep (LUSVARGHI, 1999; DI FRANCESCO, 1999).

3.3 - The relationship between allergens and dust mites.

The direct relationship between dust mite allergens in the home ecosystem and allergic diseases is corroborated by various pieces of evidence, including the fact that 60 to 80 per cent of asthma patients, including adults and children, have positive skin tests for one or more dust mite aeroallergens; bronchial provocation with dust mite extracts that trigger asthma attacks. Thus, asthma symptoms and bronchial hyperreactivity improve when individuals adopt environmental control measures to avoid these allergens (MAUNSELL et aL, 1968; PEPYS et al.., 1968; NEGREIROS et aL, 1975; PLATTS-MILLS et aL, 1992; VERVLOET et aL, 1982; CHARPIN et aL, 1988; NASPITZ et aL, 1990; EGGLESTON et aL, 1998; JULGE et aL, 1998; NISHIOKA et aL, 1998; KOVALHUK& ROSÁRIO-FILHO, 1999).

Mites secrete or excrete their products in three (3) ways: egg laying, oil secretion by glands and faecal excretion. Particles from the mite's body should not be ruled out as antigenic structures. Eggs and oil don't have allergenic properties, but faeces don't because they contain guanine, the end product of the digestion of the amino acid purine, which is one of the most important allergens in faecal contamination. So-called faecal particles represent the largest source of allergens accumulated in household dust and, because they are surrounded by a water-resistant membrane, they can remain intact for some time in the environment (SABRA & MARTINS, 1997).

Studies carried out on all continents have proven the cosmopolitan presence of *Dermatophagoides pteronyssinus,* as well as the regionalisation of other species involved in allergic processes (MAUNSELL et aL, 1968; STENIUS & CUNNINGTON, 1972; WHARTON, 1976; MUMCUOGLU, 1976; EATON etaL, 1985; FELDMAN-MUHSAM etaL, 1985; SMITH et aL, 1985; HURTADO & PARINI, 1987; CROCE et al., 1988; PARADA et al, 1988; MENDES, 1989; MALHEIROS et al, 1990; PLATTS-MILLS et al, 1992; MEDEIROS & FIGUEIREDO, 1997; GELLER, 1999).

As they are considered to have a worldwide distribution, the species of mites that most affect the population, found in the home ecosystem, are *Dermatophagoides pteronyssinus*, and, also with a wide distribution, but restricted to countries with a tropical climate, *Blomia tropicalis.* It has been shown that temperature, relative humidity and altitude have a significant influence on the acarofauna in the environment - an increase in temperature and humidity increases their density. The ideal environment for the mites to develop and breed was considered to be one with relative humidity of around 60-90 per cent and a temperature of between 20-30 °C. Under these conditions, they reproduce easily in the environment, especially in carpets, rugs, mattresses, bed linen, upholstered furniture and floor crevices; a situation mainly observed in relatively small and poorly ventilated houses, especially in winter, resulting in high indoor humidity and temperatures compatible with the development of mites (AMBROZIO et aL, 1989; MORENO et aL, 1995; VOORHORST et aL, 1969 Apud MORENO et aL, 1995).

Specifically because of the infinitely small proportions of dust mites and their droppings, which are even smaller, it has to be considered that their presence is real in practically all environments that are favourable to them, especially in terms of temperature and humidity. This makes them major triggers of allergic reactions which, due to the frequency of these reactions, lead these people to a degree of hypersensitivity due to a high concentration of IgE in the blood, causing more serious pathologies (RIZZO, 1998; MORENO et al, 1995; KONISHI & UEHARA, 1994).

Regarding the relationship between the amount of exposure to dust mite allergens and sensitisation and the onset of symptoms, studies have shown that around 2ng or 100 mites per gram of dust are enough to sensitise an individual, while around 10 Dg or 500 mites per gram of dust increase the risk of symptoms and acute asthma attacks. Other studies, however, demonstrating the importance of correlations between these arthropods and respiratory allergic diseases caused by them, state that the presence, and not a pre-established level, of allergens is sensitising (WARNER & WARNER, 1991; PLATTS-MILLS et al, 1992; MORENO et al, 1995; SABRA & MARTINS, 1997; OLIVEIRA et al, 1998; RIZZO, 1998).

In a study carried out on sensitisation to house dust mites, with both groups submitted to skin prick tests, the results, through serum IgE dosage, were positive, mainly for *Dermatophagoides pteronyssinus,* reinforcing the idea that house dust is the cause of the highest incidence of allergic conditions associated with this species of mite, and in proportion to *D. farinae* and *B. tropicalis* (OLIVEIRA et al.,1998).

In a study on sensitisation to allergens produced by mites, commonly associated with symptoms of rhinitis and bronchial asthma, of the genus *Dermatophagoides spp.* and *Blomia tropicalis,* a high prevalence of positive skin tests was observed - 96% - for *B. tropicalis,* showing a specific sensitivity to this species, which differs from the worldwide bibliography, which shows a slightly lower positivity - 60 to 78 %, leading to its inclusion in the reading skin tests. It was concluded that there seems to be a great deal of cross-sensitivity between *B. tropicalis* and *Dermatophagoides spp.* (SABRA & MARTINS, 1997).

Most asthmatic patients show immediate skin reactivity to house dust mites, with high titres of IgE, IgA and IgG against *Der p* being observed in approximately 90% of patients with positive skin tests for this species of mite, and early exposure to house dust mites plays a major role in sensitising children (RIZZO, 1998).

Along these lines, more recently, a positive response has been seen in patients with probable allergic rhinitis, negative skin tests and low total serum IgE to Dermatophagoides pteronyssinus (SOLÉ & SAKANO, 2012).

3.4 - Diagnosis of Respiratory Allergy

Several tests are available to measure IgE levels in patients' serum. Immediate reading skin tests or *Prick tests, which are* more specific than subcutaneous tests; laboratory tests, such as the RAST (RadioAllergoSorbent Test), a type of immunological test characterised by being *"in vitro"*, more specific than the *"in vivo"* test, but less sensitive (McWILL, 1999; AALBERSE.1998). The ELISA test, which is faster, simpler and more accurate, was designed to make up for the shortcomings and difficulties of previous work, seeking to control the levels of *D. pteronyssinus* and *D. farinae* antigens*, which* are the most commonly found (KONISHI & UEHARA, 1994).

Allergic manifestations are diagnosed using total serum IgE levels. In direct or collateral ancestors, these manifestations are called atopy, and are characterised by a high IgE content in the blood of these individuals. Atopy is a particular form of allergy, characterised by an increase in the immune response itself; an immediate response of violent intensity, which can trigger acute attacks of allergic rhinitis or asthma (ABBAS et al, 2000). Waldeyer's lymphatic ring, present in the nasopharyngeal region, plays an essential role in this immune response. Analysing the increase in IgE levels in total serum, at laboratory level, should be carried out together with a known positive serum and a negative serum for each batch of reagents, for a more reliable assessment of the respective levels of this specific immunoglobulin in immediate hypersensitivity reactions (ABBAS et aL, 2000; McWILL, 1999).

When inhaled allergens interact with IgE fixed on mast cells and basophils throughout the respiratory tree - the mucosa of the respiratory tract is rich in IgE - they cause the release of a variety of mediators which, together, lead to increased vascular permeability, vasodilation, contraction of bronchial and visceral smooth muscles, and local inflammation. This is known as the "immediate hypersensitivity reaction" (ABBAS et al, 2000; MALE, 1999).

Immediate Hypersensitivity Skin Tests (IHSCT) by puncture with aeroallergens are the most widely used resources in the diagnosis of respiratory allergy and show IgE-mediated allergic reactions. They have high sensitivity and specificity, comparable to "in vitro" tests for determining specific IgE (SOLÉ & SAKANO, 2012).

The importance of the proven regionalisation of the acarofauna of the home ecosystem calls attention to the re-evaluation of the antigens used to carry out immediate reading skin tests on allergic patients, which could provide information for the use of more effective desensitisation immunotherapy, based on knowledge of the species present in the geographical region where the patient lives (BROWN & FILM, 1982; GABRIEL et aL, 1985; MURRAY et aL, 1985; HURRAY et aL, 1968; BROWN & FILM, 1968). FILER, 1968; GABRIEL et aL, 1982; CUTHBERT et aL, 1984; EATON et aL, 1985; MURRAY et aL, 1985; HURTADO & PARINI, 1987; MALHEIROS et aL, 1990; SARINHO et aL, 1996; WARNER et aL, 1998; BOUSQUET et aL, 2000; EZEQUIEL, 2000).

Another test is nasal cytology, which shows the presence of eosinophils, mast cells and goblet cells in an allergic process.

3.5 - Mouth Breather Diagnosis.

A mouth breather is an individual who *"has a deviation from the normal nasal breathing pattern, usually with mouth replacement, or so-called mixed breathing; exclusive mouth breathing is rare* (QUELUZ & GIMENEZ, 2000).

In situations of nasal obstruction, one of the most frequent symptoms of allergic rhinitis, this leads to mouth breathing (MB). This occurs as a way of supplementing the small amount of air entering the lungs. As a result, the mucous membranes of the mouth and pharynx dry out, leading to irritation of the lower airways (HUNGRIA, 1995 ; RIOS, 1996).

According to QUELUZ & GIMENEZ (2000), the following types of mouth breathers are considered:

1- insufficient organic nasal breathing - mouth replacement breathing due to nasal, retronasal and oral mechanical obstacles, diagnosed clinically and radiographically;
2- insufficient functional nasal breathing - postural and functional alterations that cause mouth breathing, although there is no mechanical obstruction (allergic rhinitis);
3- functionally impotent mouth breathers - distorted pattern of breathing development due to neurological dysfunction.

The relationship between mouth breathing and malocclusion originated in studies based on the nasal/oral breathing ratio in normal children compared to long-faced children, since any disorder that occurs at the time of the formation of all this bone structure could jeopardise the respiratory system by creating situations to compensate for the body's needs, such as mouth breathing (FIELDS et al., 1991).

The effects of mouth breathing are manifested mainly on the face, where you can see a small, short nose with straight wings; the cheeks become pale and low; the mouth is constantly open; the upper lip is short; the jaw is positioned backwards and lacks development, generally shorter than normal in its length, caused by muscle pressure (CINTRA et aL, 2000; QUELUZ & GIMENEZ, 2000; LUSVARGHI, 1999; FERREI RA, 1999; DI FRANCESCO, 1999).

The relationship between mouth breathing and the relevant facial alterations is great, and there are also other important alterations in these patients, such as nocturnal apnoea syndrome, abnormal development of the thorax and hypoventilation and *cor pulmonale,* i.e. the pulmonary heart, characterised by hypertrophy of the right ventricle resulting from lung disease which, in the advanced stages, usually leads to heart failure. Elongated Face Syndrome is another important point, characterised by nasal obstruction, rhinorrhoea, sternutatory crises and nasal itching. Mouth breathing is one of the elements of information for the diagnosis of high facial angle, giving an idea of the elongation of the face (CAPELLI Jr. et aL, 2000; WHITE & PHAROAH, 2000; HIGASHI et aL, 1999; LUSVARGHI, 1999; FERREIRA, 1998; HUPPetaL, 1997; HUNGRIA, 1995; MOCELLIN,1994).

This situation tends to promote an atresia of the maxilla, i.e. a reduction in the angle formed by its arch due to the bilateral compression, in the external-internal direction, of those muscles. This compression can cause unilateral or bilateral posterior crossbite (RIOS, 1996; MARCHESAN, 1998; LUSVARGHI, 1999; QUELUZ & GIMENEZ, 2000; CINTRA et aL,2000).

ARNOLT et aL (1991), studying the relationship between RB and dental malocclusion, found that 41 (89 per cent) children of both sexes, aged between 5 and 12 years, had jaw deformities, with, among other consequences, altered dental relationships and dental malocclusions. All these children had a history of allergies.

Another consequence of the condition known as "mouth breathing" is the low amount of saliva present in the oral cavity - hyposalivation. This symptom is usually accompanied by a number of sensory changes, including changes in taste, speech and voice disorders, dysphagia and mucositis, leading to a constant need to drink fluids as a way of returning to a normal situation. Changes in the oral environment and, consequently, in the microbiota, increase susceptibility to caries. The gums, in turn, enter a process of chronic inflammation due to their dryness, leading to periodontal disease, which further aggravates the changes that make up mouth breathing (ARAGÃO, 1997; LUZ & BIRMAN, 1996; KOGA et al., 1996; MILANEZI et al., 1993).

There is no regular flow of saliva into the mouth due to the compression of the parotid duct by the buccinator muscle as it is stretched. When this saliva is released during muscle relaxation, because it has a high concentration of mucin, its viscosity increases (ARAGÃO, 1997). This increase in viscosity favours an increase in the incidence of tooth decay and, in some cases, the presence of halitosis. Salivary flow can undergo small changes, deviating from a pre-established pattern (KOGA et al., 1996; TENOVUO & LAGERLÕF, 1995; SHAFER, 1979; FIGUEIRA & NOVAES, 1997). There is a tendency to have higher salivary production, as this individual is characterised by the so-called Mouth Breather Syndrome (KOGA et al., 1996).

Extra-oral radiographs, as diagnostic aids, can suggest the occurrence of respiratory disorders. Interpreting the images provided by lateral and frontal teleradiographs is an important aid to diagnosing nasal breathing obstruction (GOMES,2000). Asymmetrical growth or progressive changes in the bone structures involved in the breathing process, according to cephalometric orientation points and planes, are points to be noted (WHITE & PHAROAH, 2000 ; HIGASHI et al.,1999; FERREIRA, 1998).

According to CINTRA et aL (2000), the success of orthodontic treatment for mouth breathers is directly linked to a good anamnesis; otherwise, there is a high chance of recurrence of malocclusion at the end of treatment.

CHAPTER 4

MATERIAL AND METHODS

This study was carried out at the Iguaçu University - UNIG, between November/2000 and May/2001. After careful examination, 32 individuals with mouth breathing associated with allergic rhinitis caused by dust mites were selected. These individuals came from private practices to hospitals belonging to the Unified Health System, on the advice of professionals; they also came from the Dental Clinic at Iguaçu University or on the suggestion/recommendation of people close to them about the way they breathe.

The stages of the work went through three phases: designing the study; collecting data and carrying out complementary tests; formatting and analysing the data.

Dentofacial morphological alterations served as a parameter for patient selection, using clinical, radiological and laboratory criteria (MARCHESAN.1998; JABUR.1998; FERREIRA, 1998;
LUSVARGHI, 1999; DI FRANCESCO, 1999; CINTRA et al.,2000; CARELLI & MIRANDA SÁ, 2001).

4.1- Preparing the study.

A predetermined sequence was followed:

- Delivery of the "Authorisation Form" for signature (Annex 1);
- Anamnesis, clinical examination and application of a questionnaire (appendix 2);
- Radiographic incidence request - P.A. (Posterior-Anterior) and Profile (appendix 3);
- Saliva collection and analysis;
- Application of immediate reading skin tests or *Prick* tests to analyse the

presence of IgE *in vivo,* specific to various antigens, including dust mites, fungi, and cockroach, dog and cat allergens.

4.2- Collecting data and carrying out complementary tests.

All the selected patients agreed to undergo these tests and evaluations by signing an "Authorisation Form" themselves or their legal guardians (appendix 1).

The aim of the data collection was to clinically identify mouth breathers by analysing the changes they have undergone over time.

At the same time, an anamnesis was taken, a clinical examination was carried out and a questionnaire was handed out (appendix 2)

4.2.1- Anamnesis

All the people who arrived for the start of the test were asked if they had any idea what mouth breathing was. From this point onwards, we sought to clarify this concept for each person and, once all doubts had been resolved, we moved on to a sequence of questions in which we sought to define the sample to be studied. The characteristics inherent to this pathology were studied, such as: mouth almost always ajar; difficulty chewing, as they find it hard to coordinate their breathing when eating; high sensitivity to external factors (e.g. household dust) causing sneezing. house dust) causing sneezing, runny nose and nasal obstruction; whether or not he slept peacefully; whether he spent a long time with his mouth open while breathing; and whether he had ever been tested to see if he really had any allergies (ARAGÃO, 1986; PLATTS-MILLS, 1987; ARNOLT et al.,1991; MOCELLIN, 1994; MARONE, 1997; MARCHESAN, 1998; FERREIRA, 1998; MERCADANTE, 1998; LUSVARGHI, 1999; QUELUZ & GIMENEZ, 2000; CARELLI & MIRANDA SÁ, 2001).

4.2.1.1- Application of the questionnaire (Appendix 2).

The aim of this questionnaire was to support the initial clinical examination for the diagnosis of mouth breathers associated with allergic pathologies.

The questionnaire sheets were distributed to the patients along with all the guidance on what it was about, in order to make the proposal clear.

The questions were addressed:

- possible sleep disturbances, such as snoring, drooling and restless sleep;
- difficulty breathing during feeding;
- presence of dry mouth and difficulty concentrating as a normal aspect;
- everyone's knowledge of whether or not they have allergies, and usually to what.

A patient who incorporated at least two of the following items was considered a "mouth breather":

-at least 1 of the sleep disorders;

-difficulty breathing while eating;

-usually have a dry mouth;

-have difficulty concentrating.

Each person's personal knowledge of having had an allergic condition served as a complementary item to be checked later.

4.2. 2-Clinical examination.

A clinical analysis showed that mouth breathers have the following main clinical characteristics. Photographs were taken in certain positions: from the front, with the individual's mouth in its usual position (ajar); and in profile, showing the convex profile of the face, according to the positioning of the jaws and lip disocclusion, in order to characterise the typical mouth breather (Figs 1 and 2).

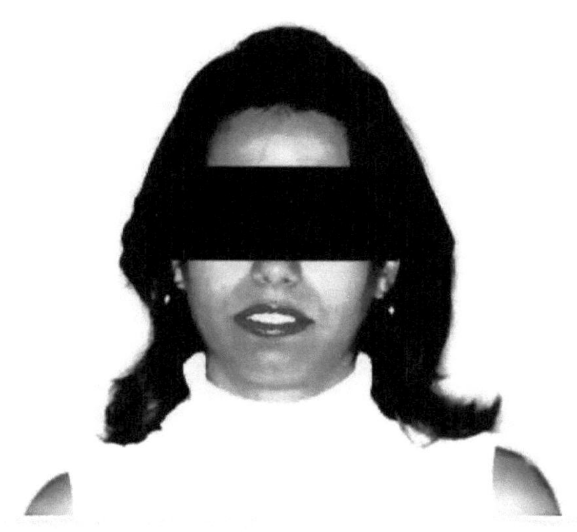

Figure 1: Photograph from the front, looking at the lip in disocclusion.

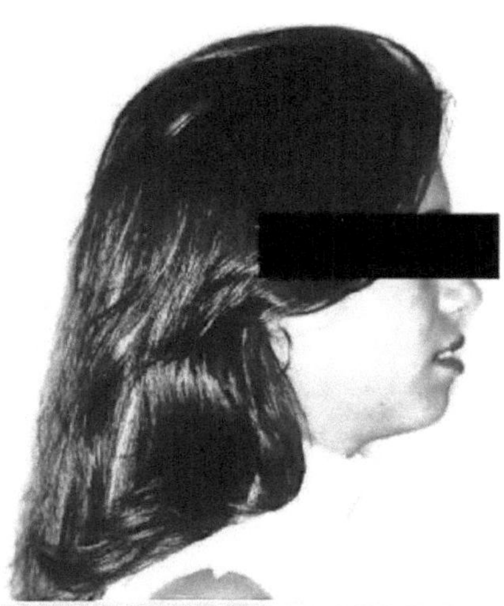

Figure 2: Profile photograph showing lip disocclusion and the convex profile of the face.

A more detailed analysis of the oral cavity revealed an ogival palate (Fig. 3), caused by muscle pressure, especially the buccinator and masseter, which are stretched and compress the jaw.

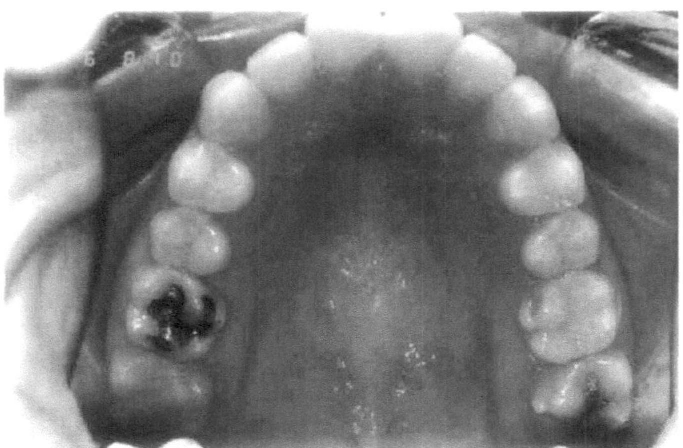

Figura 3: Photograph of the palate, showing its deepening.

Facial analysis, which is the analysis of facial measurements taken directly from the patient during the clinical examination, has recently come back into use as an auxiliary means of analysing facial aesthetics. The proportion between the width and height of the face, the so-called facial index, seeks to establish the overall facial type of each individual (PROFFIT, 1995).

Facial Anthropometric Measurements - (in mm)

Parameters	Male	Standard deviation	Female	Standard deviation
Height of the lower third of the face	72	6,0	66	4,5
Gonial width	97	5,8	91	5,9

Table 1: anthropometric measurements in young adults (adapted from PROFFIT, 1995)

Mouth breathers were those who presented as such in at least one (1) of the items: anamnesis or clinical examination.

4.2.3- Radiological examination

In order to establish a correct diagnosis of the origin of predominantly mouth breathing, due to bone malformation or trauma, or due to allergic conditions. Each patient was asked to undergo radiological examinations. Of the scans, two were chosen because it was relatively easy to find a service that would perform them, and also because these scans were sufficient to help form a correct diagnosis. These are Postero-Anterior (P.A.) and Lateral Profile (PROFFIT,1995; FERREIRA, 1998).

The aim was to isolate mouth breathers with a different cause, such as an anatomical alteration alone, from those with the characteristics of mouth breathers of allergic origin, the subject of this study.

Orientation points and plans were observed for the Mouth Breather:

1- deviated septum - important as a cause of mouth breathing;
2- apical displacement of the palatine vault - marked or not;

By correlating this data with the 'Facial Anthropometric Measurements' (Table 1), a more accurate analysis of each case can be obtained.

The 'Measurements' are as follows, taken in the P.A. incidence: i-gonial distance - (or bigonychial distance) - from gonion to gonion of the mandible, in a straight horizontal line (correlated to the measurement taken directly on the patient using the curved callipers);

3- height of the lower third of the face - from the base of the nose (ENA-superior -- anterior-superior nasal spine) in a straight vertical line, to the chin.

According to GUIMARÃES NETO et al. (1998), the mustachioed distance is a cephalometric reference for a study subject to minimal errors, due to the stability of its position, making it possible to reproduce it faithfully by means of measurements carried out by the computer after its manual localisation.

	Lower facial height (ENA-Me)			
	Male		Female	
Age group (years)	Average value	Standard deviation	Average value	Standard deviation
6	59	3,6	57	3,2
9	62	4,3	60	3,6
12	64	4,6	62	4,4
14	68	5,2	64	4,4
16	71	5,7	65	4,7

Table 2: Harvold Standard Values (mm), study from 6 to 16 years (adapted from PROFFIT, 1995)

Because of the proportionality of the measurements used for the height of the lower third of the face, its method has been proven with age and mandibular growth, and also according to the stable localisation characteristic of this reference (GUIMARÃES NETO et aL, 1998), this proportionality of growth could be applied to this measurement, as shown in table 3.

	Bigoniac distance			
	Male		Female	
Age groups	Average value	Standard deviation	Average value	Standard deviation
6	74	7,1	73	5,2
9	88	6,8	84	5,0
12	97	6,8	91	5,0
14	97	6,4	91	4,9
16	97	6,2	91	4,8

Table 3: Values considered standard for bigonaca distance (mm).
(as per PROFFIT, 1995)

A cephalometric analysis provides a tracing that allows us to visualise the bone changes that have occurred. These changes can lead to other changes, such as dental ones, aggravating the initial problem. Mouth breathers, due to the alteration in the breathing process, have these changes more markedly (FERREIRA, 1998; PROFFIT, 1995).

According to FERREIRA (1998), cephalometry is a method that obtains linear and angular measurements of the various anatomical elements of the skull and face. The 'Computerised Cephalometric Analysis', with its respective tracing, was carried out by Dr[3] . Cláudia Maria Romano de Souza, a specialist in Radiology, using the RADIOCEF programme - version 2.0, manufactured by Radiomemory.

We used the Sassouni Analysis criteria (PROFFIT, 1995), in which the vertical and horizontal relationships, and the interaction between these proportions, reflect a vertical proportionality of the face through the so-called Horizontal Anatomical Planes (Fig. 4), as termed by Sassouni. In well-proportioned faces, these planes tend to converge at a single point, showing a balance of the face. A rotation of the maxilla downwards in the posterior region and upwards in the anterior region brings about the anticipated intersection of the palatal, occlusal and mandibular planes. This results in facial proportions that are long in the anterior region and short posteriorly, predisposing to an open bite malocclusion. The so-called "adenoid face", characteristic of mouth breathers, consists of narrow widths, protruding teeth and lips with some separation (QUELUZ & GIMENEZ, 2000; SILVA et al., 2000; PROFFIT, 1995).

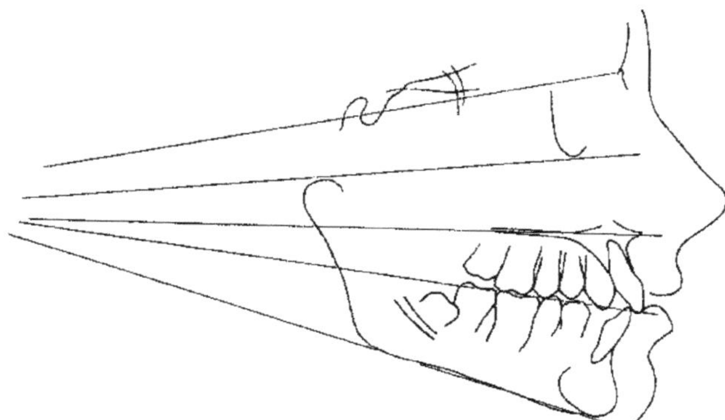

Figure 4: Sassouni Cephalometric Planes

The Plans studied in Sassouni's analysis, presented in the following order, from highest to lowest, are:

- Inclination of the anterior cranial base

  (nasion point in the centre of the sella turcica)
- Frankfurt plan
- palatal plane
- occlusal plane
- mandibular plane

In the P.A. incidence, alterations in the structures of the nasal region were analysed, such as septal deviations. The impairment of nasal breathing due to obstruction in the region, which is largely responsible for mouth breathing, would consequently exclude that patient, as it is beyond the scope of this study. Patients with structural alterations in the maxillary sinuses due to chronic infections, such as sinusitis, hindering the normal breathing process, were also excluded from this study (CHACONAS, 1987; VION, 1994; PROFFIT, 1995; FERREIRA, 1998).

In the Lateral Profile view, the aim is to demonstrate the convex profile normally found in mouth breathers; the degree of deepening of the anterior palate - or hard palate, in relation to the positioning of the incisals of the upper central incisors, comparing these with the cusp tips of the upper 1^{oS} premolars, both in a straight vertical line towards the palate. The position of the anterior teeth is also altered, with an increase in the distance between the dental arches (overjet), retrusion of the mandible and postural protrusion of the maxilla, resulting in the protrusion of these anterior teeth (CHACONAS, 1987; FIELDS etaL, 1991; VION, 1994; PROFFIT, 1995; FERREIRA, 1998). These measurements were adopted because there is no single standard of measurement that allows the palate to be studied separately and its depth in mouth breathers. A value of 2.0 cm was used as a reference measurement, and above this is considered to be a marked degree of deepening of the palate, characterising the mouth breather.

Patients with a change in one of the items were considered positive:

- gonial distance shorter than the measurement considered standard;
- height of the lower 1/3 of the face greater than the measurement considered standard;
- presence of apical displacement in the palatine vault.

4.2.4 - Salivary collection and analysis

The collection of stimulated saliva gives us the opportunity to measure the amount produced by the salivary glands at a predetermined time. There are various methods used for this purpose, and saliva was collected according to the Cury technique, which uses the DentoBuff® salivary analysis kit (INODON, 1988) (Fig. 5).The following salivary analysis provided an additional parameter, since the oral cavity suffers directly from changes in the individual's natural profile (QUELUZ & GIMENEZ, 2000; SILVA et al, 2000;

FIGUEIRA Jr. & NOVAES, 1997; LUZ & BIRMAN, 1996; KOGA et al, 1996; THYLSTRUP & FEJERSKOV, 1995; SHAFER et al. 1979), 1979).This analysis consists of 2 tests:

- the salivary flow rate: the values corresponding to salivary flow were measured in millilitres per minute (ml/min), according to the recommended technique (FIGUEIRA Jr & NOVAES, 1997; TENOVUO & LAGERLÕF, 1995).
- the buffering capacity of saliva: measured on a scale from 3.0 to 7.0 (INODON, 1988), according to which it ranges from a low to a high capacity to neutralise pH changes that occur at certain times in the oral cavity.

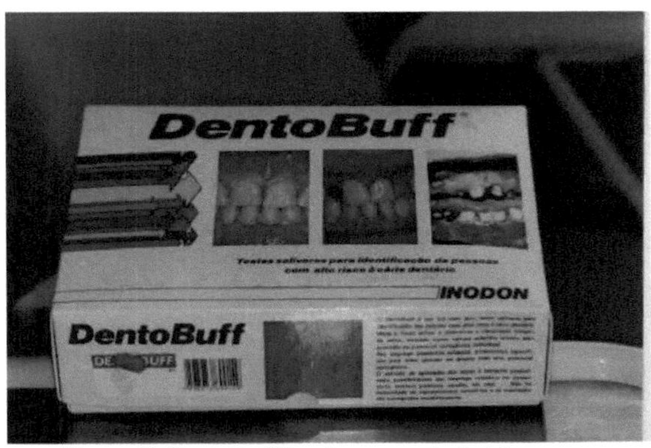

Figure 5: DentoBuff® salivary analysis kit.

The two tests were based on standardised scales (Fig. 6 ; Fig. 8) respective.

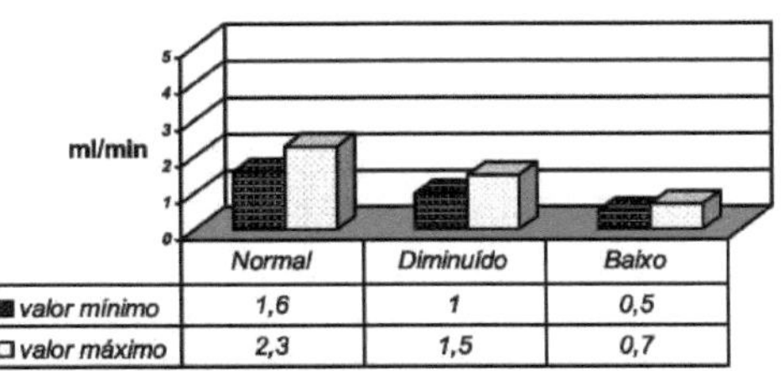

Figure 6: Average salivary production values, considered as standard, collected using the stimulated saliva technique.

The following technique was used to check the salivary flow rate:

- the subject had to be fasting for 2 hours before the procedure;
- chew a gum base tablet to stimulate salivary secretion (Fig. 7);
- during the gum softening process, the saliva was completely discarded;
- From then on, the timekeeping of
  2 minutes, with the patient continuing to chew the gum;
- During this period, all the saliva produced was collected in a previously prepared container (Fig. 7);
- At the end of this time, the volume produced was noted, disregarding the foam on the surface;
- the final volume was obtained using a graduated pipette, divided by the time used by the patient (ml/min);

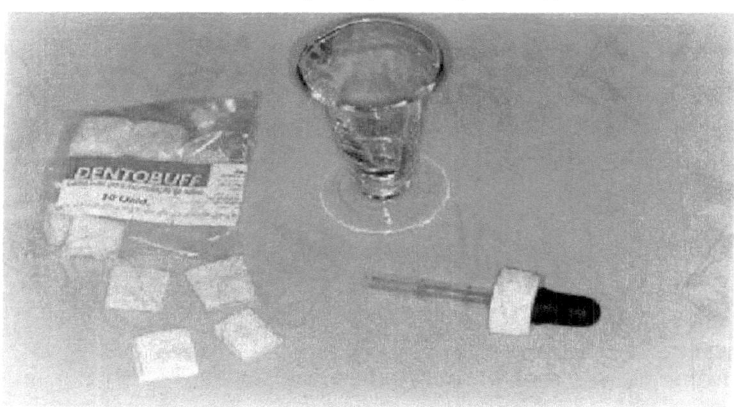

Figure 7: Material used for stimulation and saliva collection.

The same saliva collected underwent another type of test, the "Salivary Buffer Capacity", which analyses the ability of saliva, when faced with pH changes in the oral cavity, to always seek a return to equilibrium, based on predetermined values considered.

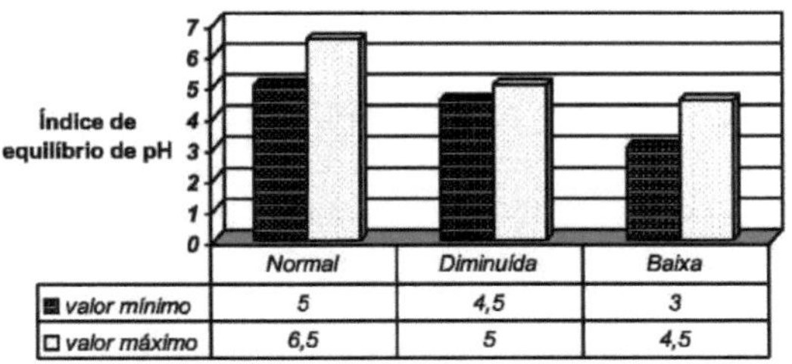

	Normal	Diminuída	Baixa
■ valor mínimo	5	4,5	3
□ valor máximo	6,5	5	4,5

Figure 8: Standardised mean values for salivary buffer capacity.

The results of this test are analysed using a colorimetric scale provided by the manufacturer. Based on the results obtained using this scale, saliva has a normal, intermediate or low ability to seek a pH rebalance after feeding and the start of digestion in the oral cavity (Table 4).

To check the buffering capacity of the saliva, now that the patient was not present, the following technique was used:

- 1ml of the saliva collected from the patient was removed from the respective container using a graduated pipette, keeping it in an upright position, and the saliva was poured into a previously prepared flacon containing an acidic solution;
- 4 drops of an indicator solution were added;
- The flacon was capped and shaken for about 10 seconds to homogenise;
- The lid was removed and left to stand for 5 to 10 minutes, then closed again;
- The colour of the mixture was compared with the Kit's colour scale;
- According to the colour, a numerical value was obtained on the scale that indicates from low buffering capacity to normality.

This is a way of quantifying an individual's cariogenic potential. It should be noted that a person's cariogenic potential must be assessed in conjunction with other variables: general health, type of diet and oral hygiene habits, to name a few.

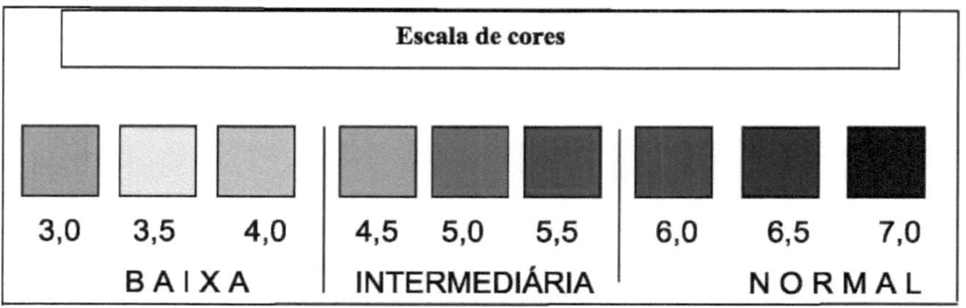

Chart 4: Colour scale for defining Salivary Buffer Capacity (adapted from Inodon do Brasil - Kit DentoBuff ®).

4.2.5- Immediate reading skin tests or *Prick test*.

In order to determine the allergic cause, in addition to an anamnesis and the application of an individual questionnaire, "*Prick* tests" were also carried out as a way of analysing these patients' responses to various inhaled antigens, in an attempt to confirm the presence of Gell & Coombs type I hypersensitivity.

These tests were carried out by ProP. DP. Oscarina da Silva Ezequiel, an allergist and professor at the Federal University of Juiz de Fora - MG.

As well as limiting this allergic condition to dust mites, a profile was drawn up of the different allergens that could also cause it.

The procedure for the epicutaneous test comprises defined and ordered steps in order to control the expected result (ALI, 1993; EMERSON & CORDEIRO, 1993).

In simple terms, the steps were ordered as follows:

- A battery of standardised tests has been established, according to what is being researched;
- The site of application of all the extracts was defined for each patient, in a pre-established sequence;

- The patient was instructed not to touch the area during the test;
- the reading was taken, looking for the parameter of the reaction caused by the histamine.

The allergens used were: house dust; extracts from 3 species of mites *(Dermatophagoides pteronyssinus, Dermatophagoides farinae and Blomia tropicalis),* extracts from 2 groups of fungi, group 1 (made up of *Alternaria alternata , Chaetomium globosum*) and group 3 (made up of *Aspergillus fumigatus , Penicillium notatum, Alternaria alternata*); as well as allergens from cockroaches *(Blatella germanica),* dogs *(Canis familiaris)* and cats *(Felis domesticas).* A negative control with saline solution and a positive control with histamine at a concentration of 10 mg/ml were used. All the allergenic extracts came from the same source - the IPI-ASAC laboratory in Brazil.

The application was made on the inside of the right forearm in all patients in order to have a standardised study and analysis; and always in the same local application sequence. The reading was taken 20 minutes after the application in each patient, comparing the extent of the reaction to each allergen with the positive (histamine) and negative (saline) controls. The positive and negative controls were used as an evaluation parameter. The degree of sensitivity to any of the allergen extracts was analysed in relation to the degree of sensitivity to histamine, as well as the occurrence of sensitivity to saline solution. The aim was to avoid false-positive and false-negative results.

The degree of skin positivity was measured using the modified Pepys criterion, where the intensity of the reaction was assessed using crosses (+). The answers obtained represented the sensitivity, specificity, precision and relevance of the test (EMERSON & CORDEIRO, 1993):

(+) → the papule formed is larger than 3 (three) mm, but smaller than the histamine reactive papule;

(++) → the papule formed with the same diameter as the histamine papule;

(+++) → the papule formed with a larger diameter than the papule formed by histamine;

(++++) → in addition to the larger diameter of the papule formed in relation to

to the histamine papule, pseudopodia were formed, demonstrating much greater sensitivity.

4.3- Data formatting.

The data from the tests used in this study were tabulated and analysed separately using graphs. This format provided a general assessment of mouth breathers and their association with dust mites as the main agents causing allergic problems.

4.4- Statistical treatment and analysis of the data obtained.

By comparing the various tests used in this study, we sought to establish the relationship between mouth breathing and hypersensitivity with the induction of allergic rhinitis, specifically to house dust mites, and the oral alterations resulting from this condition, examined over a wide age range, from 3 years old to 53 years old, placing house dust mites as the most important indirect cause of these alterations, given the rate at which they were found.

After each test was carried out to characterise the mouth breather, a diagnosis was made specifying the cause. Correlation tests and chance-risk tests were carried out to quantify the potential for mite antigens to induce mouth breathing.

CHAPTER 5

RESULTS

After the initial examinations, the cephalometric analysis of the Profile and P.A., the salivary flow assessment and the hypersensitivity skin tests, the following results were obtained.

1) Anamnesis, clinical examination and answers to the questionnaire.

Of the 40 individuals examined according to the characteristic signs (e.g. mouth almost always ajar, difficulty in maintaining breathing through the nose), 32 of them (80 %) were selected in addition to the known anthropometric standards (table 1). After analysing the anamnesis and clinical examination together, eight patients were excluded because they had no visual alterations or anthropometric measurements that met the proposed requirements. The answers given by only the selected patients, classified in Table 5, sought to show the profile of patients considered to be mouth breathers.

		Sleep disturbances			While eating		Normally					
Patient No.	**Age**	snoring	Babar	be agitated	Can breathe		Do you have a dry mouth?		Difficulty concentrating?		Do you know	
											aiert	liar
					S	N	S	N	S	N	S	N
01	**03**			X		X	X			X	X	
02	**04**	X		X		X		X		X	X	
03	**10**	X		X	X		X		X		X	
04	**10**		X	X	X		X			X	X	
05	**14**	X	X			X	X			X		X
06	**16**		X	X	X		X			X	X	
07	**16**		X	X		X	X		X		X	
08	**18**	X	X	X	X		X		X		X	
09	**20**		X	X	X		X		X		X	
10	**20**	X	X	X	X		X		X		X	
11	**20**		X		X			X	X		X	
12	**21**		X		X		X			X	X	
13	**21**	X		X	X			X	X		X	
14	**21**		X		X		X		X			X
15	**22**	X	X	X		X		X	X		X	
16	**22**		X	X	X		X		X		X	
17	**22**		X		X			X		X	X	
18	**23**		X	X	X			X	X		X	
19	**23**		X		X			X	X			X
20	**29**		X		X			X		X		X

21	**30**	X		X		X	X			X	X	
22	**30**	X	X		X		X			X	X	
23	**31**	X			X		X			X	X	
24	**32**					X		X	X		X	
25	**37**		X			X		X	X		X	
26	**38**	X			X		X		X		X	
27	**39**	X	X	X	X		X		X		X	
28	**40**		X			X		X	X		X	
29	**41**	X		X	X		X		X		X	
30	**44**	X		X	X		X		X			X
31	**50**	X		X		X	X		X		X	
32	**53**				X			X		X	X	

Chart 5: Clinical mouth breathers' responses to the questionnaire, according to age.

Analysing the answers to the questionnaire applied to the 32 patients selected, after anamnesis and clinical examination, revealed that, according to the pre-established criteria, all the patients could be considered mouth breathers. After analysing the answers to the questionnaire, it can be seen that in the 21 to 30 age group, the age group with the largest number of patients, practically all of them reported the presence of some or all of these disturbances. There was also a higher proportion (72.73 %) between the patients examined in this age group (total=11) and those who believed they had allergies (total=8) (Fig. 9).

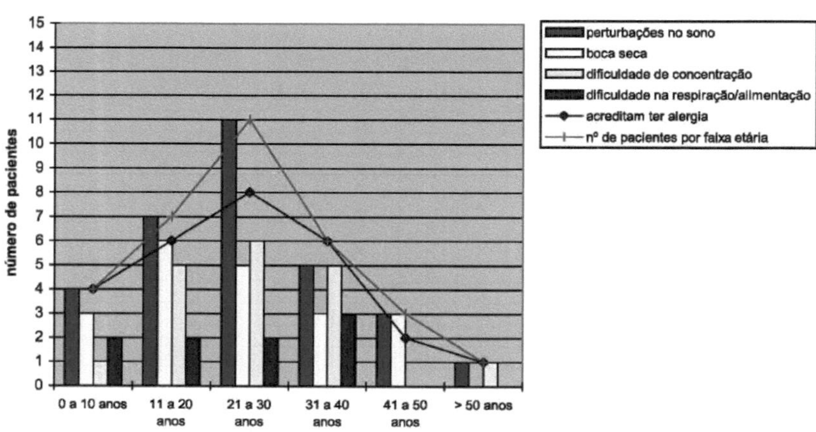

Figure 9: Number of patients considered to be mouth breathers by answers to the questionnaire, according to age group.

Among the allergenic factors known to the patients and reported in the same questionnaire, house dust played an important role, being present in practically all age groups. The

Mites were reported in the 0 to 10 age group, with a coincidence of proportions with house dust. Fungi, as inducers of allergic responses, were reported at a higher rate in the 31 to 40 age group (Fig. 10).Mouth breathers were patients who presented themselves as such in at least one of the items: anamnesis or clinical examination.

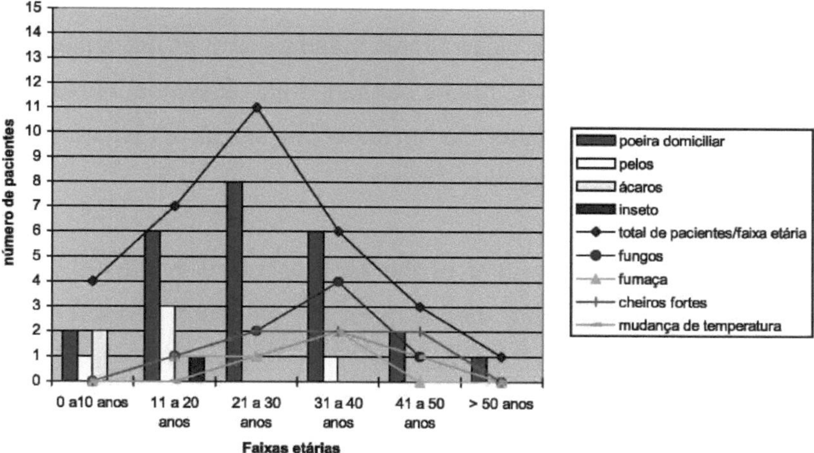

Figure 10: Number of patients considered to be mouth breathers due to factors that trigger or exacerbate allergy symptoms, according to age group.

The item 'smoke' was described by the patients as smoke from cigarettes, car exhausts and fires.

The item 'strong smells' was described as perfumes, disinfectants and room flavourings, coinciding with the item 'smoke' and the item 'fungus' in the first two age groups (0-10; 11-20). In the next age group (21-30), the items 'strong odours' and 'fungus' only coincided.

The item 'change in temperature' was described as a change in climate to a colder temperature, as well as being associated with relative humidity, coinciding with the item 'fungi' in the last two age groups studied (41-50; >50).

2) X-ray examination.

Since there is a tendency for mouth breathers to have an elongated face, due to changes in reference parameters such as the gonial distance and the height of the lower third of the face, we have that (chart 6):

- Goniac distance less than the established standard did not occur in any of the patients examined; however, there were values that, although above the standard, were close to this standard in 3 of the patients - 9.37% - who had their radiographs subsequently examined. However, the gonial distance parameter did not show any significant alteration in terms of characterising mouth breathers.

- Enlargement of the lower third of the face occurred in 29 (90.62%) patients; changes of more than 20% of the standard measurement occurred in 11 (34.37%) patients.

Patient No.	Age	Deviated septum		Goniac distance (mm)		Height of the lower 1/3 of the face (mm)		Palatine vault (apical displacement)	
		S	N	standard	Enc.	Standard	Enc.	S	N
01	**03**	X		73	80	54	59	X	
02	**04**		X	75	88	56	70		X
03	**10**		X	84	105	62	71	X	
04	**10**		X	82	100	60	70		X
				average	**93,25**		**67,50**		
05	**14**		X	91	102	68	70		X
06	**16**		X	91	100	65	70	X	
07	**16**		X	91	110	65	90	X	
08	**18**		X	91	100	66	55	X	
09	**20**		X	91	105	66	68	X	
10	**20**		X	91	114	66	78		X
11	**20**		X	97	115	72	75		X
				average	**106,57**		**72,29**		
12	**21**		X	91	105	66	78	X	
13	**21**		X	91	110	66	65		X

14	**21**		X	91	100	66	75	X	
15	**22**		X	91	95	66	75	X	
16	**22**		X	91	110	66	70	X	
17	**22**		X	91	110	66	83		X
18	**23**		X	97	115	72	75		X
19	**23**		X	91	118	66	80		X
20	**29**	X		91	103	66	80	X	
21	**30**		X	91	98	66	78	X	
22	**30**		X	91	105	66	85	X	
				average	**106,27**		**76,73**		
23	**31**		X	**91**	105	66	80		X
24	**32**		X	91	100	66	85	X	
25	**37**	X		91	110	66	95		X
26	**38**		X	97	110	72	70	X	
27	**39**	X		**91**	108	66	75	X	
28	**40**		X	91	105	66	85	X	
				average	**106,33**		**81,67**		
29	**41**		X	91	115	66	75	X	
30	**44**		X	91	100	66	70		X
31	**50**		X	91	108	66	80	X	
				average	107,67		75		
32	**53**		X	91	98	66	78	X	
					98		78		

Chart 6: Radiographic analysis of mouth-breathing patients studied, according to age.
Legend: standard = standard measure
Enc. = measurement found on the patient

In the study of the radiographic views of these patients, alterations were observed in certain points of the skull, the so-called Craniometric Points, in relation to the standard measurements for those used as a reference to prove mouth breathing (FIELDS etal., 1991).

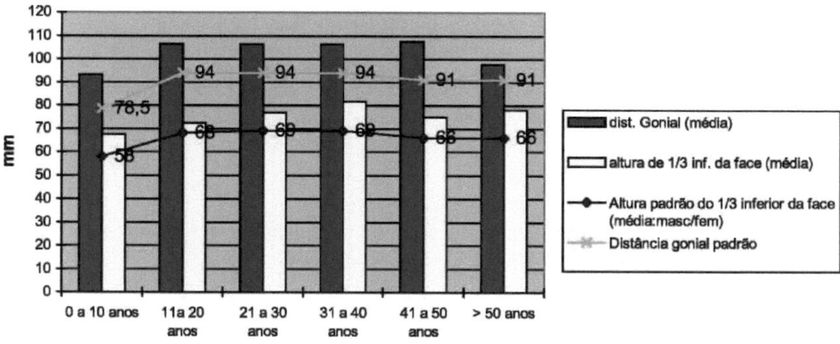

Figure 11: Average gonial distance and average height of the lower third of the face (mm) of the mouth breathers examined, according to age group.

The gonial distance found in the patients was unchanged,

corresponding to a value lower than the standard. With regard to the measurement of the lower third of the face, changes were observed in all age groups, emphasising that in the 0 to 10 age group, there were major changes, since this is precisely the period of greatest growth and bone development (Fig. 11).

The discrepancies between the values found for the gonial distance and the height of the lower third of the face were analysed separately, showing the age groups where the greatest standard deviations occurred (Figs 12 and 13). The greatest standard deviation occurred in the 11 to 20 age group for the lower third of the face height parameter.

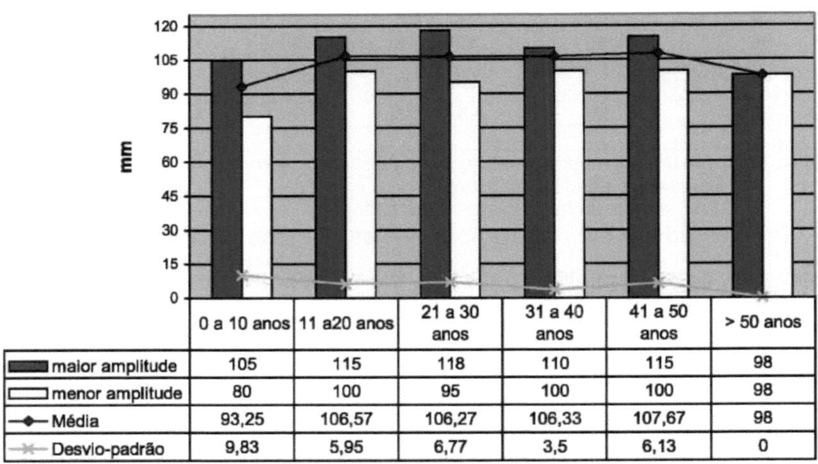

	0 a 10 anos	11 a20 anos	21 a 30 anos	31 a 40 anos	41 a 50 anos	> 50 anos
maior amplitude	105	115	118	110	115	98
menor amplitude	80	100	95	100	100	98
Média	93,25	106,57	106,27	106,33	107,67	98
Desvio-padrão	9,83	5,95	6,77	3,5	6,13	0

Figura 12: Measures of Central Tendency and Dispersion of the Gonial Distance (mm) of the Mouth Breathers examined, according to age group

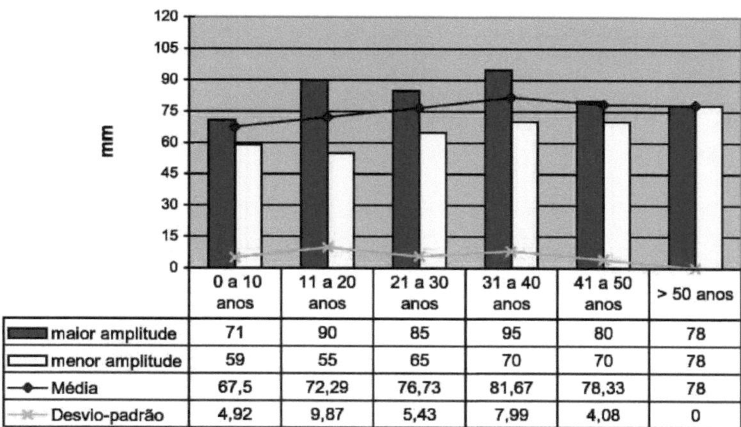

	0 a 10 anos	11 a 20 anos	21 a 30 anos	31 a 40 anos	41 a 50 anos	> 50 anos
maior amplitude	71	90	85	95	80	78
menor amplitude	59	55	65	70	70	78
Média	67,5	72,29	76,73	81,67	78,33	78
Desvio-padrão	4,92	9,87	5,43	7,99	4,08	0

Figura 13: Measures of Central Tendency and Dispersion of the Height of the Lower 1/3 of the Face of Mouth Breathers Examined, According to Age Group.

Patient 13 was excluded because he didn't show any significant changes for Mouth Breathing in any of the 3 items considered, resulting in 31 patients being analysed, although he was included within the criteria adopted in the anamnesis and clinical examination. Radiological examination revealed no tumours or bone malformations that could induce mouth breathing.

In the study population, four patients had a small deviated septum, which was not considered an important factor in nasal obstruction.

Palate deepening occurred in 20 (62.50 %) of the patients, according to the lateral profile radiographic view (Fig. 14).

Of the 29 patients who presented with enlargement of the lower third of the face, the following were observed:

- 6 patients (20.68%) had a more marked deepening of the palate, coinciding with the 11 patients who had alterations greater than 20%;

- 12 patients (41.37%) had a deepened palate;

- 11 patients (37.93%) did not have a deepened palate.

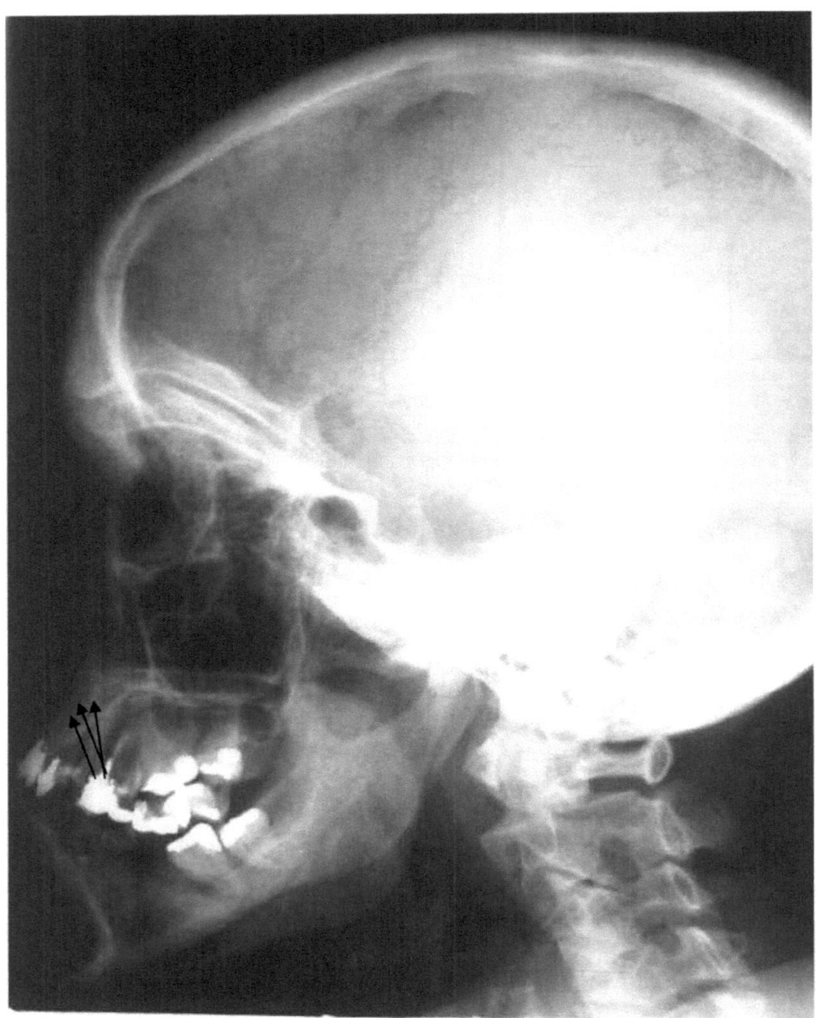

Figure 14 - Lateral profile X-ray showing the characteristic appearance of deepening of the palate (arrows).

3) Salivary analysis.

Table 7 shows the values obtained for each patient. With regard to salivary flow, saliva was collected in a graduated vial after being stimulated, according to the established technique (Fig. 15). The highest concentration was found in the intermediate range, where there may be a tendency towards oral pathologies due to some alteration in the saliva, regardless of age group.

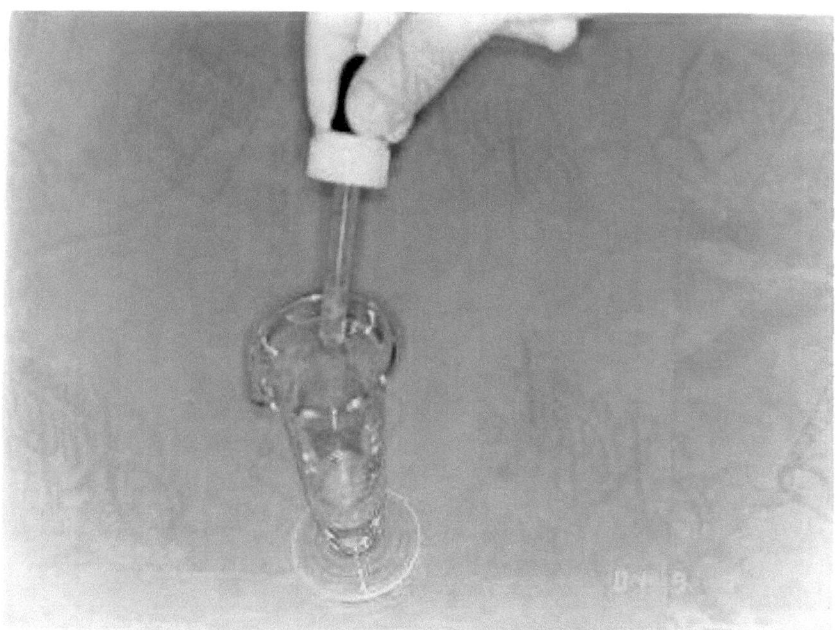

Figura 15: Saliva collected at the end of the programmed time, followed by examination of the buffer capacity.

With regard to Buffer Capacity, the highest percentage of patients had a low buffer capacity, i.e. a low ability to neutralise changes in oral pH (Fig. 16).

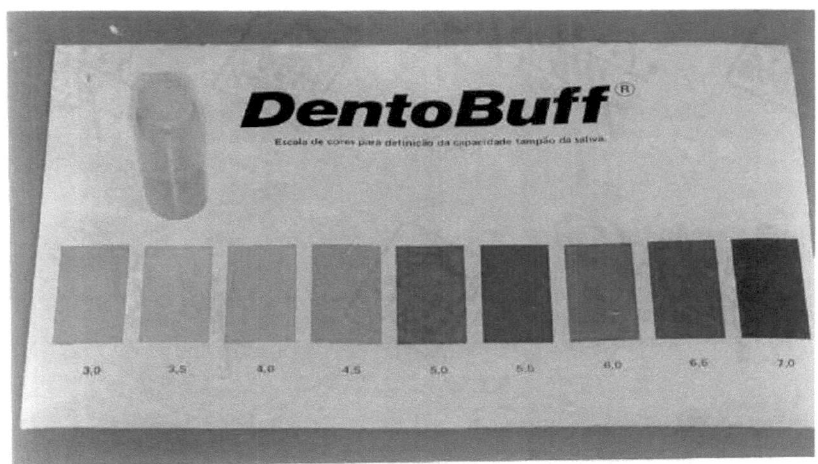

Figure 16: Evaluation of the buffering capacity of saliva in a collected sample and the respective scale.

3.0 to 4.0 - low
4.5 to 5.5 - intermediate
6.0 to 7.0 - normal

Patient No.	Age	Salivary flow (ml/min)	Average By age group	Buffer Capacity	Average By age group
01	**03**	1,5		4,0	
02	**04**	0,5		6,5	
03	**10**	1,25		3,5	
04	**10**	1,5	1,19	3,5	4,38
05	**14**	1,25		3,5	
06	**16**	1,0		4,5	
07	**16**	2,0		3,5	
08	**18**	0,75		3,5	
09	**20**	1,75		5,5	
10	**20**	1,5		3,5	
11	**20**	1,25	1,36	3,5	3,93
12	**21**	1,5		3,5	
13	**21**	1,25		3,5	
14	**21**	3,0		3,5	
15	**22**	1,25		4,5	
16	**22**	1,0		4,0	
17	**22**	2,25		3,5	
18	**23**	1,25		4,0	
19	**23**	2,0		3,5	
20	**29**	2,35		6,5	
21	**30**	2,5		4,5	
22	**30**	1,75	1,83	3,5	4,05
23	**31**	3,0		3,5	
24	**32**	2,75		4,5	
25	**37**	1,5		4,0	
26	**38**	1,75		3,5	
27	**39**	1,75		4,5	
28	**40**	3,25	2,33	3,5	3,92
29	**41**	2,0		4,0	
30	**44**	2,25		3,5	
31	**50**	1,75	2,00	3,5	3,67
32	**53**	1,5	1,50	5,0	5,00

Chart 7: Saliva flow and buffer capacity of mouth-breathing patients studied, according to age.

The two tests analysed together showed that in mouth-breathing patients, saliva is altered to such an extent that it leads to the appearance of other pathologies (e.g. caries and periodontal disease), aggravating the initial condition. Of a total of 31 patients, since patient 13 had already been excluded after a negative radiological examination for the alterations investigated, only 2 (6.45 %) had no alterations in Flow and Buffer Capacity; and 15 patients (46.87 %) had both alterations. The average values, tabulated in figure 17, allow us to analyse the samples collected against the standard values already mentioned.

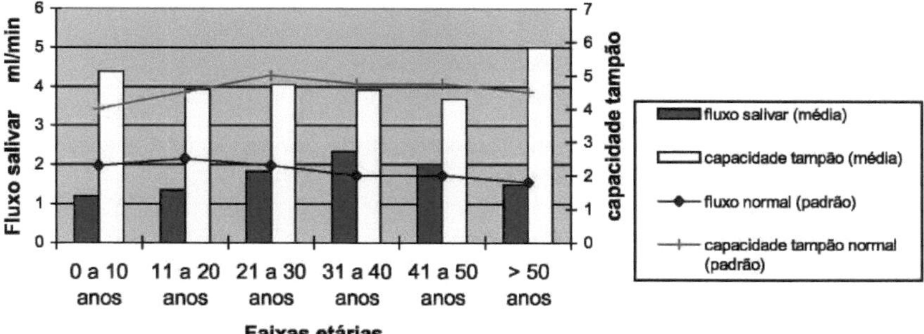

Figure 17: Mean values for saliva flow and buffer capacity of the mouth breathers studied, according to age group.

Next, the variations in salivary flow and buffer capacity were analysed in isolation. It was observed that the increase in flow occurred in direct relation to age, up to the age of 40, and then began to decrease (Fig. 18).

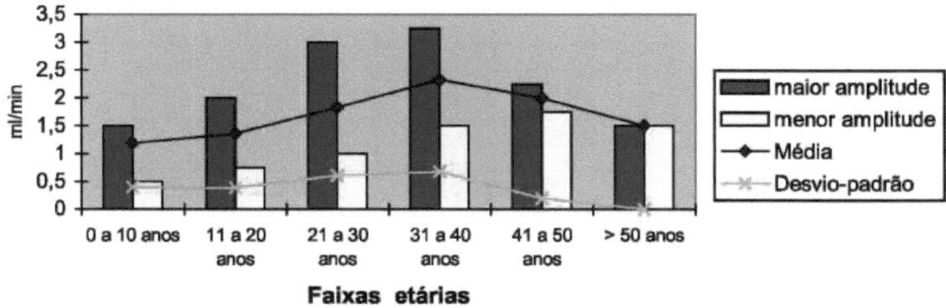

Figure 18: Measures of Central Tendency and Dispersion of Salivary Flow of the mouth breathers studied, according to age group.

With regard to Buffer Capacity (Fig. 19), it was observed that in almost all age groups it was around 3.5, a value considered critical for the onset of secondary pathologies.

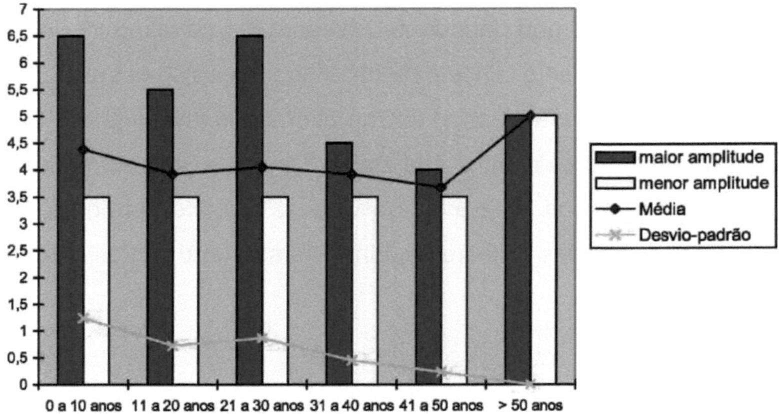

Figure 19: Measures of Central Tendency and Dispersion of the Salivary Buffer Capacity of the mouth breathers studied, according to age group.

4) Immediate reading skin tests - Prick test.

The following table (table 8) lists the respective tests and the degree of sensitivity of each patient to the antigens applied.

			Acaras			Fungi		Other antigens			negative control	Positive control
Patient No.	**Age**	House dust	*D.p.*	*D.f.*	*B. t.*	grp1	grp3	cheap	dog	cat	Saline solution	Histamine (10mg/ml)
01	**03**	-	-	-	-	-	-	-	-	-	-	Yes
02	**04**	-	++++	-	-	-	-	-	-	-	-	yes
03	**10**	-	+++	-	-	-	-	-	-	-	-	yes
04	**10**	-	-	-	-	-	-	-	-	-	-	yes
05	**14**	+	+++	-	-	-	-	-	-	-	-	yes
06	**16**	+	++	++	-	-	-	-	-	-	-	yes
07	**16**	-	+	+	-	-	-	-	-	-	-	yes
08	**18**	-	+++	-	-	-	-	-	-	-	-	yes
09	**20**	+	++	+	++++	++++	-	-	-	-	-	yes
10	**20**	+++	++	-	+++	-	-	-	-	-	-	yes
11	**20**	+	-	-	-	-	-	-	-	-	-	yes
12	**21**	+++	++++	+++	+++	+++	-	-	+	-	-	yes
13	**21**	-	-	-	-	-	-	-	-	-	-	yes
14	**21**	+	-	-	-	-	-	-	-	-	-	yes
15	**22**	+	++++	++++	-	-	-	-	-	-	-	yes
16	**22**	+	+++	++	-	++	-	+	-	-	-	yes
17	**22**	++++	++++	+++	+++	-	-	-	-	-	-	yes
18	**23**	+++	++++	-	-	-	+	-	-	-	-	yes
19	**23**	+	-	-	-	-	-	-	-	-	-	yes
20	**29**	+	-	-	-	-	-	-	-	-	-	yes
21	**30**	-	+	-	-	-	-	-	-	-	-	yes
22	**30**	++	++++	++++	+	+	-	-	-	-	-	yes

23	**31**	+	-	-	-	-	-	-	-	-	-	yes
24	**32**	+	++++	+++	+++	+	+	-	+	-	-	yes
25	**37**	-	+	+	+	-	-	-	-	-	-	yes
26	**38**	++	++++	++++	++++	-	-	+	-	-	-	yes
27	**39**	-	-	-	-	-	-	-	-	-	-	yes
28	**40**	++++	++++	++++	+	-	-	-	-	-	-	yes
29	**41**	+	-	-	-	-	-	-	-	-	-	yes
30	**44**	-	-	-	-	-	-	-	-	-	-	yes
31	**50**	-	-	-	-	-	-	-	-	-	-	yes
32	**53**	+++	+++	+++	-	-	-	-	-	-	-	yes

-egenda: next Legend:

house dust - house dust
D. p. - Dermatophagoides pteronyssinus
D. f. - Dermatophagoides farinae
B. t. - Blomia tropicalis

(-) - no result
(+) - degree of positivity, according to the modified Pepys scale

Fungi: grp *1-A. alternata* and *C. globosum*
grp 3- *A. fumigatus, P. notatum* and *A. alternata* cockroach *(Blatella germanica);* dog *(Canis familiaris);* cat *(Felis domesticus).*

Chart 8: Immediate Reading Skin Tests or *Prick-Test,* in the mouth-breathing patients studied, according to age.

Positive and negative controls were used to define possible false-positive and false-negative reactions.

In the results of these tests, each patient was analysed separately, showing the following:

Patient 1: 3 years old, negative tests, which could be false negative due to the age group. In these cases, we can't say whether it's an allergy or not, we rely on the clinical history and family history. Therefore, this patient was considered allergic, without defining the cause.

Patient2: Patient with allergic rhinitis with positive tests for *D.pteronyssinus* exclusively and significantly.

Patient3: Patient with allergic rhinitis with positive tests for *D.pteronyssinus* exclusively and significantly.

Patient 4: Patient with non-allergic rhinitis with negative tests at an age with little chance of false negatives.

Patient 5: Patient with allergic rhinitis who tested positive for *D. pteronyssinus* and house dust, the latter of which we considered positive despite its lower intensity.

Patient 6: Patient with allergic rhinitis who tested positive for *D. pteronyssinus, D. farinae* and house dust.

Patient 7: Patient with allergic rhinitis with positive tests, although weakly positive for *D. pteronyssinus and D. farinae.*

Patient 8: Patient with allergic rhinitis, according to positive test results for *D. pteronyssinus* exclusively and significantly.

Patient 9: Patient with allergic rhinitis with a significant presence of positive tests for *D. pteronyssinus, B. tropicalis, D. farinae,* house dust and fungi; the most significant being for *B. tropicalis* and intra-house fungi (the latter is an uncommon finding, as skin tests for fungi are not usually found to be very positive).

Patient 10: Patient with allergic rhinitis who tested positive mainly for *B. tropicalis and* house dust, but to a lesser extent for *D. pteronyssinus.*

Patient 11: Patient with allergic rhinitis and weakly positive tests for house dust.

Patient 12: Patient with allergic rhinitis who tested significantly positive for house dust, *D. pteronyssinus, D. farinae, B. tropicalis and intra-house fungi, as* well as dog.

Patient 13: Patient with non-allergic rhinitis with negative tests at an age with little chance of false negatives.

Patient 14: Patient with allergic rhinitis and weakly positive tests for house dust.

Patient 15: Patient with allergic rhinitis who tested significantly positive for *D. pteronyssinus and D. farinae, and* to a lesser extent, but also positive, for house dust.

Patient 16: Patient with allergic rhinitis presenting positive tests for multiple antigens: house dust (weak), *D. pteronyssinus, D. farinae,* intra-house fungi, cockroach.

Patient 17: Patient with allergic rhinitis who tested significantly positive for house dust, *D. pteronyssinus, D. farinae* and *B. tropicalis.*

Patient 18: Patient with allergic rhinitis who tested significantly positive for house dust and *D. pteronyssinus.*

Patient 19: Patient with allergic rhinitis and weakly positive tests for house dust.

Patient 20: Patient with allergic rhinitis and weakly positive tests for house dust.

Patient 21: Patient with allergic rhinitis and weakly positive tests for *D. pteronyssinus.*

Patient 22: Patient with allergic rhinitis who tested significantly positive for *D. pteronyssinus, D. farinae and* to a lesser extent for house dust, *B. tropicalis* and intra-house fungi.

Patient 23: Patient with allergic rhinitis and weakly positive tests for house dust.

Patient 24: Patient with allergic rhinitis who tested significantly positive for *D. pteronyssinus, D. farinae* and *B. tropicalis*, to a lesser extent for house dust, intra-house fungi from groups 1 and 3, as well as the dog.

Patient 25: Patient with allergic rhinitis and weakly positive tests for *D. pteronyssinus, D. farinae* and *B. tropicalis.*

Patient 26: Patient with allergic rhinitis who tested significantly positive for *D. pteronyssinus, D. farinae* and *B. tropicalis;* to a lesser extent for house dust and cockroaches.

Patient 27: Patient with non-allergic rhinitis with negative tests at an age with little chance of false negatives

Patient 28: Patient with allergic rhinitis who tested significantly positive for house dust, *D. pteronyssinus* and *D. farinae* and, to a lesser extent, for *B. tropicalis.*

Patient 29: Patient with allergic rhinitis and weakly positive tests for house dust.

Patient 30: Patient with non-allergic rhinitis with negative tests at an age with little chance of false negatives.

Patient 31: Patient with non-allergic rhinitis with negative tests at an age with little chance of false negatives.

Patient 32: Patient with allergic rhinitis who tested significantly positive for house dust, *D. pteronyssinus and D. farinae.*

Figures 20 and 21 illustrate the skin reactions presented, to varying degrees, by the patients who underwent the skin tests.

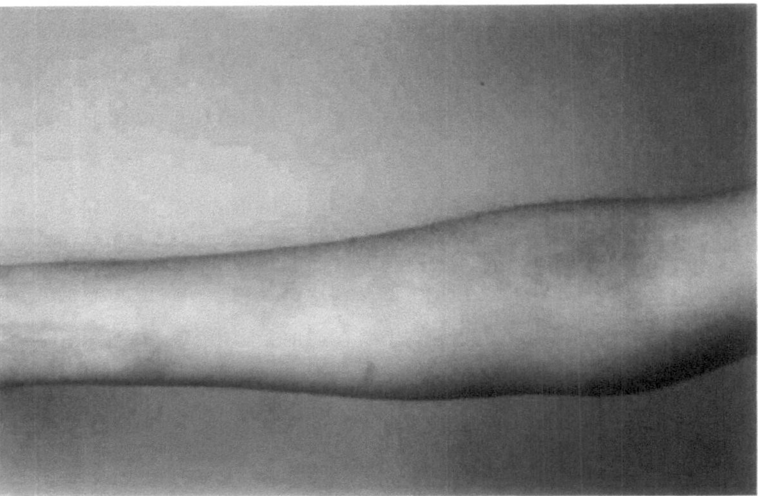

Figure 20: Example of skin reaction after application of allergen extracts presented by patients.

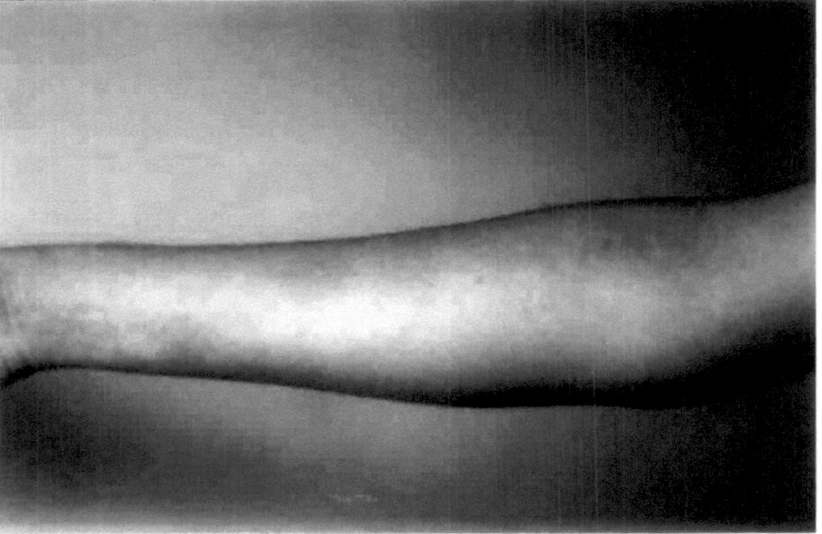

Figure 21: Another example of the patient's reaction.

It was observed that mites were present in almost all age groups, with *D. pteronyssinus* being the most constant species, showing high reactivity compared to the number of patients examined (Fig. 22).

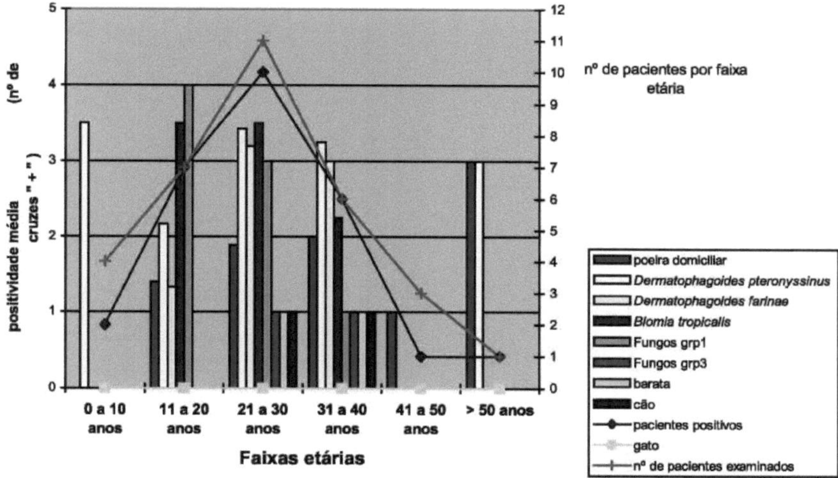

Figure 22: Average positivity of mouth breathers examined for different allergens, according to age group.

In the relationship between house dust and mites, *D. pteronyssinus* was again found to be a constant, *although* it does show that other mite species are also important (Fig. 23).

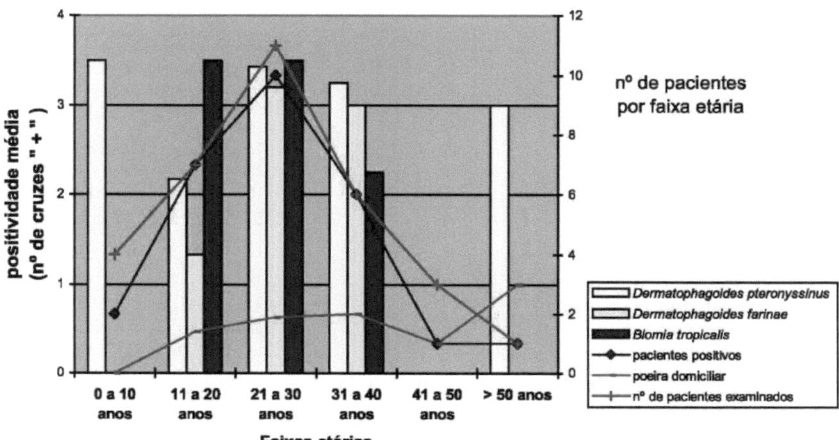

Figure 23: Average positivity of mouth breathers for dust mite and house dust allergens, according to age group.

Analysing the sensitivity to house dust showed an increase in direct proportion to age, with a sharp drop in the 41 to 50 age group and then high sensitivity in the following age group (Fig. 24).

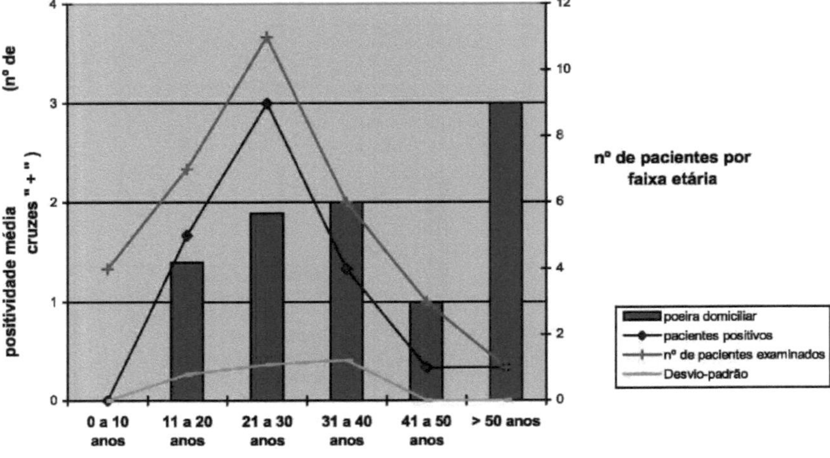

Figure 24: Sensitivity to house dust

The data evaluated in Fig. 25 shows the sensitivity to the most common mites according to the respective age group, and the *D. pteronyssinus* species proved to be constant, while there was also a high sensitivity to *B. tropicalis.*

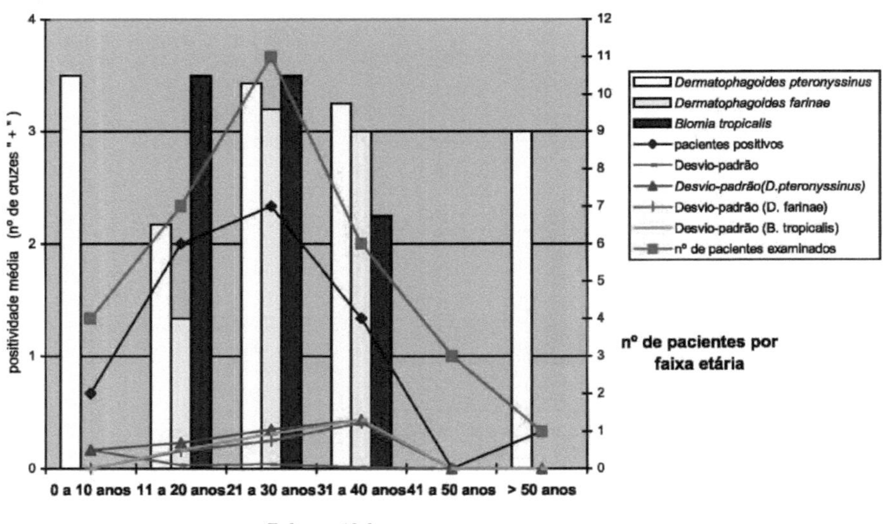

Figure 25: Sensitivity to the most common mites

In a first analysis, 31 patients were examined, excluding patient no. 13, where high positivity was found in the 11 to 20 and 21 to 30 age groups. When analysing positivity exclusively for mites, patient number 1 was excluded as it was not possible to know the specific cause of the reaction obtained (Table 1).

Table 1: Variations in positivity to specific antigens

Age group	Patients examined		Positive Patients		Ag positive patients - mites		Ag-positive patients - dust		Ag-positive patients - fungi		Ag - positive patients	
	N°	%	N°	%	N°	%	N°	%	N°	%	N°	%
0-10	04	12,90	02	50	*02	66,67	0	00	0	00	0	00
11-20	07	22,58	07	100	06	85,71	05	71,43	01	14,29	0	00
21-30	10	32,26	10	100	07	70	09	90	04	40	02	20
31-40	06	19,35	05	83,33	04	66,67	04	66,67	01	16,67	02	33,33
41-50	03	9,68	01	33,33	0	00	01	33,33	0	00	0	00
>50	01	3,23	01	100	01	100	01	100	0	00	0	00
TOTAL	31	100	26	83,87	*20	66,67	20	66,67	06	20	04	13,33

Caption:

* 1 patient in the 0-10 age group was excluded from this analysis because it was considered a false negative.

Ag= Antigen

The Odds Ratio test showed, with a 95% confidence interval, that the chances of a patient with allergic rhinitis caused by dust mites developing Mouth Breathing are very high. This result was corroborated by Spearman's Correlation Test which, based on the adapted Rugg table, showed a correlation considered to be high (table 9).

"ODDS RATIO.

Data	Sample 1	Sample 2	
Success	20	6	-
Failures	0	4	-
Results:			
Odds Ratio"=	13,3333	-	-
(P)=	0,0487	-	-
95% CI=	1,	2418<= μ<=143	

	,1574

Caption:

(p) = probability of error

CI = Confidence Interval

Successes = mouth-breathing patients

Failures = non-mouth-breathing patients

Sample 1 = mite-sensitive

Sample 2 = not sensitive to mites, but to other sources.

"PEAR MAN CORRELATION"

Correlation Coefficient	0,8986

Table 9: Results of the tests carried out.

CHAPTER 6

DISCUSSION

Mouth breathing, according to Angle (1907) apud CINTRA et al. (2000), *"is the most powerful cause, constant and varied in its results, causing the so-called -bad-occlusions and an asymmetrical development of the facial muscles linked to the process itself, leading to a disorganisation of the functions performed by the lips, cheeks and tongue. Its main cause is nasal obstruction*

Evaluating the entire picture of the patients involved showed that each one was interested in knowing that the problem existed and what the probable cause was. The most commonly confirmed concern was aesthetics and, secondarily, chewing and speech. Socially, the individual's acceptance into the environment and society is linked to preconceptions such as aesthetics, phonetics and diction. This is portrayed in a picture of facial disharmony, occlusal disharmony, with consequences mainly for speech and mastication (MARCHESAN, 1998; MOCELLIN,1994), situations that meet the functional needs of each individual.

The anamneses, together with the clinical examinations, served as a basis for constructing the universe of patients who were subsequently assessed in more detail, since the clinical signs of mouth breathers are very characteristic.

Errors in phonetic pronunciation are often associated with dental alterations, predominantly mouth breathing and early tooth loss, leading children to have difficulties with certain phonemes. Observing the number, shape and inclination of the teeth and whether or not they have cavities is important when first analysing the patient. A different number of teeth in the lower arch compared to the upper arch will probably result in a deviation from the midline, with the appearance of larger spaces between the teeth, which will tend to be occupied by the more posterior teeth in a mesialisation movement, altering the original uniform distribution of these teeth in the arches, hence the importance of an early diagnosis of the condition, for treatment with more positive results (MARCHESAN.1993; CARELLI & MIRANDA SÁ, 2001).

As a diagnostic aid, extra-oral radiographs can suggest the occurrence of respiratory disorders by detecting, for example, asymmetrical growth or progressive changes in the bone structures involved in the breathing process. Mouth breathing is believed to be one of the elements of information for analysing the high facial angle, which is formed by two cephalometric orientation planes - the Frankfurt Plane and the Mandibular Plane. This primary study of the patient gives an idea of the increase in the face, which is then complemented by other points and planes of cephalometric orientation to arrive at the height of the lower third of the face, better localising the problem (CAPELLI Jr. et aL, 2000; WHITE & PHAROAH, 2000 ; HIGASHI et aL, 1999; FERREIRA, 1998).

Ratifying the importance of saliva in the formation and development of caries lesions, the main factors involved in this process were listed: tooth factor, saliva factor and diet factor (SHAFER et al, 1979). This led to the conclusion that the amount of salivary flow, i.e. the volume of saliva produced over a predetermined period, is considered the most important clinical parameter for analysing mouth breathers, significantly affecting their susceptibility to caries lesions on tooth surfaces (FIGUEIRA & NOVAES, 1999; THYSLTRUP & FEJERSKOV, 1995; TENOVUO & LAGERLÕF, 1995). Salivary flow, characterised as a local examination, showed that mouth breathers had a higher average salivary flow, and noticeably more viscous, which would cause an increase in the rate of caries and periodontal disease (KOGA et aL , 1996 and ARAGÃO, W., 1997).

The analysis of the allergic process in the mouth-breathing patients analysed was based above all on the results obtained, after a previous pathological history of atopy, asthma and even atopic dermatitis had been ruled out during the selection process.

The greater or lesser intensity of the tests does not necessarily imply a greater or lesser degree of allergy, in the sense of the severity of the symptoms, but rather the potential to develop responses that end up altering the normal respiratory mechanism.

When it comes to correlating orofacial alterations with dust mite allergy, especially in terms of the relationship between the individual and the age group, there is a consensus in the literature that the earlier the onset of breathing difficulties due to allergy, the easier it is for bone and dental alterations to occur and their consequences for the individual, such as low ventilatory capacity (LUSVARGHI,1999;DI FRANCESCO,1999;FERREIRA,1999; QUELUZ & GIMENEZ, 2000; CAPELLI et al, 2000). This can be seen from the evaluation tabulated in figures 11, 12 and 13, where mites were always present as inducers of allergic response, some species more than others and more constant, as was the case with *D. pteronyssinus* , clearly demonstrating the relationship between mite antigens and the level of induction of Mouth Breathing. House dust is of great importance in this analysis, as it serves as a substrate for mite proliferation, associated with temperature and humidity characteristics.

Before 1960, certain habits in children were considered normal, such as playing outside, walking or cycling. However, in the years since, changes in habits have taken hold and a more sedentary lifestyle has led people to considerably reduce their frequency of physical activity. There is a possibility that this sedentary lifestyle may have contributed to an increase in bronchial reactivity, since people, being constantly indoors, do not have the necessary air renewal, presenting a higher concentration of suspended materials than is considered normal (RIZZO.1998; MORENO et al.,1995). Exposure to indoor and outdoor air pollutants has been recognised as a potential risk for the development and exacerbation of respiratory diseases. Intra-household pollutants are associated with cigarette smoke and the infiltration of particulate matter suspended in the air (e.g. combustion products, the vaporisation of pesticides and carbon monoxide [CO], which in overcrowded urban areas has its concentration dispersed in the air increased). Household dust is also seen as a factor responsible for allergic conditions, as it is a mixture of organic and inorganic substances (e.g. dog, cat and rabbit hair and epithelium, fungi, insects and dust mites) (RIZZO,1998; MORENO et al.,1995).

Immediate hypersensitivity skin tests are easy to perform and are a great help in the etiological diagnosis of allergic conditions. The literature mentions that children at the age of three show a reaction to histamine 61% of the diameter of adults (FORTE et al., 2001), and that false negatives can also occur. Studies indicate that positivity to different allergens suggests that skin tests below the age of four would not be as valuable, as they are less positive in children up to the age of four, reaching greater positivity from adolescence to young adulthood, followed by a decline with age (FORTE et al., 2001).

Skin tests are an excellent contribution and are considered the primary diagnostic resource for confirming immediate hypersensitivity, as they demonstrate the presence of specific IgE antibodies to the antigens investigated, helping to identify the allergens responsible for the condition, since it is multifactorial. Immunological reactions for specific IgE may be more suitable than skin tests in some situations, mainly for assessing cross-reactions, and because the reactivity of dermal tests in children up to three years old is usually low (AALBERSE.1998).

The indications for RAST IgE testing are skin lesions that prevent the immediate reading skin test from being carried out, such as atopic dermatitis associated with rhinitis and asthma; as well as the use of antihistamine drugs that would promote a false-negative response.

Despite the development of methods for detecting IgE antibodies *"in vitro"*, immediate reading skin tests, carefully carried out with potent antigens and positive and negative control substances, are still the most revealing procedures for diagnosing specific allergic factors associated with allergic rhinitis. Direct skin tests with the appropriate allergens are the fastest and least expensive, making them an important aid in the aetiological diagnosis of atopy (PAHO, 1989; AMBROZIO et al, 1989; FORTE et al, 2001; ALI, 1993; EMERSON & CORDEIRO, 1993). It is essential that the results are examined in relation to the patient's current problems with a direct correlation with the clinical history both with skin tests and *"in vitro"* techniques (PAHO, 1989; ALI, 1993).

The majority of serums that react to *D. pteronyssinus* will also react to extracts of storage mites. This is largely due to the cross-reactivity that can exist, as in the results obtained in figures 19, 20 and 22 (AALBERSE, 1998; SABRA & MARTINS, 1997).

The possibility of this evidence was observed through the RAST test, showing that the D. *pteronyssinus* extract was the most efficient inhibitor, and thus the most likely inducer of IgE stimulation (AALBERSE, 1998). False-positive reactions can occur when the substance is in high concentration, when the test was carried out on an area where the skin was previously irritated or eczematised or when the vehicle used in the contact test is irritating for that patient. False-negative reactions can occur when the concentration of the allergen is low, when the vehicle used is unsuitable, when the test is withdrawn for a shorter period of time than indicated or when the test is carried out in an area where topical corticosteroids have been used for less than a week, and especially the use of systemic antihistamines (ALI, 1993); factors that were observed and strictly complied with, including the suitability of the laboratory that manufactured the extracts. Even so, we had one patient, number 1 (one), who presented a false negative result, which could be interpreted as such due to his age group; the diagnosis was based on the child's clinical history - allergic without a defined cause.

CHAPTER 7

CONCLUSIONS

The correlation between RB and hypersensitivity associated with the mite is as follows:

This correlation is high, with a marked risk of the allergic individual becoming a mouth breather when they come into contact with the mite.

The mite species found most frequently in the different age groups was *D. pteronyssinus.*

The increase in factors triggering allergic symptoms was directly proportional to the number of patients examined, with house dust as a constant allergen. Of the 26 patients considered to be mouth breathers, 20 (76.92 %) were for dust mites.

Salivary analysis of the patients showed a joint alteration in flow and buffer capacity in 15 (48.39 %) patients, indicating the need for greater care of the oral cavity in patients who are proven mouth breathers.

In the cephalometric analysis, the measurement of the lower third of the face provided technical and precise information, showing alterations in all age groups, with the lower age groups being the ones most in need of care so as not to permanently install mouth breathing, with the consequent alterations.

Public health programmes must control dust mites in the home environment, with the aim of building affordable housing with good ventilation, avoiding an environment favourable to dust mite proliferation.

Public health programmes that provide conditions for the early diagnosis, treatment and prophylaxis of mouth breathers, with multidisciplinary monitoring, are necessary in order to avoid more serious anatomical and organic alterations, especially in children during periods of bone development.

CHAPTER 8

BIBLIOGRAPHICAL REFERENCES

AALBERSE, R. C. 1998. Allergens from mites: implications of cross-reactivity between invertebrate antigens. **Allergy, 53** (Suppl 48): 47-48.

ABBAS, A. K.; LICHTMAN, A. H.; POBER, J.S. 2000. **Cellular & Molecular Immunology.** 3ª ed. Editora Revinter. Rio de Janeiro, p. 210-214; 271-280; 306-320.

ALI, S.A. 1993. Epicutaneous Tests, Contact Tests or Patch Tests. Why use and how to use. **Rev. Bras. Allerg. Imunopatol.,** 16(5): 192-197.

AMBROZIO.L.C.; BAGGIO,D.; MORIJ.C.; FERNANDES, M.F.M.; KASE, M.T.; MELLO, J.F. 1989. *Suidasia pontifícia', a* respiratory tract allergiser? Preliminary investigation of antigens from other genera of house dust mites. **Rev. Bras. Allerg. Immunol.,** 12(1): 15-23.

ANDRADE, Z.A.; LENZI, H.L.; LENZI, J. 1991. Pathological processes caused by parasitism; regeneration and healing. Chap. 8:94-103 In **Parasitologia** (Rey, L. org.). 2ª ed. Editora Guanabara-Koogan. Rio de Janeiro. XXVIII+ 731 pp.

ARAGÃO.W. 1986. Mouth breathers (MB). **Odontol.** Mod. ,13(7):39-41.

ARAGÃO, W.1997.The saliva of the mouth breather. **J. bras. Odontol. Clin.,** 1(1):65-67.

ARNOLT, R.G.; DAGUERRE, N.; SERRANI, J. C.; VIGNAU, S. 1991. The mouth breather and dental-maxillary changes. **Archiv. Argent. Allerg. Immunol. Clin., 22(2):84-87.**

BERNARD, PH. 1986. Nasal obstruction and rhinorrhoea. Chap. 6:69-73. in: **How to recognise, understand and treat frequent pathological conditions in Otorhinolaryngology.**
BERNARD,PH.;FERRON,P.;NARCY,PH.;HUY,P.T.B.;
UZIEL, A. Organ. Andrei Editora Ltda. São Paulo. 395 pp.

BERND, L.A.G.; BAGGIO, D.; BECKER, A.B.; AMBROZIO, L.C. 1994. Identification and study of the sensitising activity of house dust mites in Porto Alegre (RS). **Rev. Bras. Allerg. Imunopatol.**, 17:23-33.

BOUSQUET, J.; LOCKEY, R.F.; MALLING, H.J. 2000. Allergen immunotherapy: therapeutic vaccines for allergic diseases. Report from the World Health Organisation. **Rev. Bras. Allerg. Imunopatol.,** 23:1-55.

BROWN, H.M. & FILER, J.L. 1968. Role of mites in allergy to house dust. **Br.** Med. J., 3:646-647.

CAPELLI Jr. J. ; CARLINI, M.G. ;OLIVEIRA, S.R. 2000. Facial Growth and the Treatment of Anterior Open Bite. **Rev. Bras. Odontol., 57(2):76-** 79.

CARELLI, E.G. & MIRANDA SÁ, M. O. S. 2001. Phonetic analysis in patients with dental alterations. **Rev. Fono Atual,** 15:39-42.

CHACONAS, S. J. 1987. Classification of malocclusion. Chap.2:15-33; Radiographic Cephalometry. Chap.3:35-92 In **Orthodontics.** 1ª ed. Guanabara-Koogan. Rio de Janeiro. Livraria Editora Santos. São Paulo.

CHARPIN, D.; KLEISBAUER, J.P.; LANTEAUME, A.; RAZZOUK, H.; VERVLOET, D. 1988. Asthma and allergy to house-dust mites in populations living in high altitudes. **Chest,** 93(4):758-761.

CINTRA, C.F.S.C.; CASTRO, F. F. M.; CINTRA, P. P. V. C. 2000. Orofacial alterations in mouth-breathing patients. **Rev. Bras. Allerg. Imunopatol., 23(2):78-83.**

COHEN, S.R. 1980. *Cleyletiella dermatitis.* A mite infestation of rabbit, cat, dog and man. **Arch. Dermatol.,** 116:435-437.

COLOFF, M.J. 1998. Taxonomy and Identification of dust mites. **Allergy,** 53(suppl 48):7-12.

BRAZILIAN CONSENSUS ON ASTHMA MANAGEMENT, II° .1998. **J. Pneumol., 24(4):** 176-177;197-201.

CROCE, P.M.; BAGGIO, D.; CROCE, J. 1988. House dust mites in Lima, Peru. **Rev. Bras. Allerg. Imunopatol., 11** (5): 179. Abs 122.

CUTHBERT, O.D.; BROSTOFF, J.; WRAITH, D.G.; BRIGHTON, W.D. 1979. "Barn allergy: asthma and rhinitis due to storage mites. **Clin. Allergy,** 9:229-236.

DI FRANCESCO, R. C. 1999. Mouth breathers: the otorhinolaryngologist's view. **J. Bras. Ortod. Ortop. Facial, 4** (21):241-247.

EATON, K.K.; DOWNING, F.S.; GRIFFITHS, D.A.; LYNCH, S.; HOCKLAND, S.; McNULTY, D.W. 1985. Storage mites culturing, sampling technique, Identification and their role In house dust allergy In rural areas In the United Kingdom. **Ann. Allergy,** 55:62-67.

EGGLESTON, P.A.; ROSENSTREICH, D.; LYNN, H.; GERGEN, P.; BAKER, D.; KATTAN, M.; MORTIMER, K.M.; MICHELL, H.; OWNBY, D.; SLAVING,

R.; MALVEAUX, F. 1998. Relationship of indoor allergen exposure to skin test sensitivity in inner-city children with asthma. **J. Allergy Clin. ImmunoL,** 102:563-570.

EMERSON, M.F.E. & CORDEIRO, N.G.B. 1993. Mouth breathing in children with allergic rhinitis: the tip of an iceberg. **Rev. Soc. Bras. Allerg. ImunoL, 16(2):51-64.**

EZEQUIEL. O.S. 2000. **Evaluation of the acarofauna of the domiciliary ecosystem in the municipality of Juiz de Fora, state of Minas Gerais, Brazil.** Master's thesis in Parasitic Biology. FIOCRUZ. Oswaldo Cruz Institute. xv+77p.il.

FACCINI, J.L.H.; SERRA-FREIRE, N.M.; MELLO, R.P. 1991. Acari: The ticks, chap.60: 650-657 In **Parasitologia** (Rey, L. org.). 2ª ed. Editora Guanabara-Koogan. Rio de Janeiro. XXVIII + 731 pp.

FACCINI, J.L.H.; SERRA-FREIRE, N.M.; MELLO, R.P.; GALVÃO, A.B. 1991. Acari: The mites of scabies and other dermatoses. ch.61: 657-661 In **Parasitologia** (Rey, L. org.). 2ª ed. Editora Guanabara-Koogan. Rio de Janeiro. XXVIII + 731 pp.

FAIN, A.; GUÉRIN, B.; HART, B.J. 1990. **Mites and Allergic Disease.** Allerbio. Varennes en Argonne, 190p.

FELDMAN-MUHSAM, B.; MUNCUOGLU, Y.; OSTEROVICH, T. 1985. A survey of house dust mites (Acari: Pyroglyphidae and Cheyletidae) in Israel. **J. Med. Entomol.,** 22:663-669.

FERREIRA, F.V. 1998. Diagnosis and Clinical Planning. Chap. 22:475- 501 In **Orthodontics. Diagnóstico e Planejamento Clínico.(FERREIRA,** F.V.

org.). 2ª ed. Artes Médicas Publishing House. São Paulo.

FERREIRA, M. L. 1999. The incidence of mouth breathers in individuals with Class II occlusion. **J. Bras. Ortod. Ortop. Facial,** 4(21):224-239.

FIELDS, H.W. ; WARREN, D.W. ; BLACK, K. ; PHILLIPS,C. 1991. Relationship between vertical dentofacial morphology and respiration in adolescents. **Am. J. Orthod. Dentofac. Orthop.,** 99:147-154.

FIGUEIRA Jr., E. & NOVAES, F. R. 1997. Important aspects in the study of saliva. **Rev. Faculd. Odontol. Valença,1** (1): 36-39.

FORTE, W.C.N.; CARVALHO Jr.,F.F.; FERNANDES F[lo] ., W.D.; SHIBATA,E.; HENRIQUES, L.S.; MASTROTI,R.A.; GUEDES, M.S. 2001. Immediate hypersensitivity skin tests with advancing age. **J. Pediatr. (Rio J.), 77(2):** 112-118.

FRANKLAND, A.W. & EL-HEFNY, A. 1971. House dust and mites as causes of inhalant allergic problems in the United Arab Republic. **Clin. Allergy,** 1:257-260.

FRIEDLAENDER, M.H. 1996. Allergic disorders of the eye. In BIERMAN, C.W. & PEARMAN, D.S. **Allergy, Asthma and Immunology from infancy to adulthood.** 3ª ed. WB Saunders Company, Philadelphia. p. 703-712.

GABRIEL, M.; CUNNINGTON, A.M.; ALLAN, W.G.L.; PICKERING, C.A.C.; WRAITH, D.G. 1982. Mite allergy in Hong Kong. **Clin. Allergy, 12:157-** 171.

GALVÃO, A.B. & GUITTON, N. 1986. House dust mites in Brazilian capitals and Fernando de Noronha Island. **Mem. Inst. Oswaldo Cruz, 81** (4):417-

430.

GELLER, M. 1990. Respiratory atopy in Rio de Janeiro. **Ann. Allergy,** 64:171-173.

GELLER, M.; ESCH, R.E.; FERNÁNDEZ-CALDAS, E. 1995. *Euroglyphus mainey* sensitisation in patients with respiratory atopy in Rio de Janeiro. **Rev. Bras. Allerg. Imunopatol.,** 18(6):215-218.

GELLER, M. 1996. Dust mite allergy in Rio de Janeiro. **J. Bras. Medic.,** 71(1/2): 12-14.

. 1999. An OverView of mite allergy in Brazil **Cad. Allerg. Asthma Immunol.,** 11(2):17-22.

GOMES, D.C. 1991. Main groups of protozoan and metazoan parasites of man and their vectors. Chap. 9:104-112 In **Parasitologia** (Rey, L. org.). 2ª ed. Editora Guanabara-Koogan. Rio de Janeiro. XXVIII + 731 pp.

GOMES, M.A. 2000. Study of the airways using lateral and frontal teleradiographs. **Rev. Assoe. Asso. Radiol. Odontol., 1(1):** 15-19.

GUIMARÃES NETO, R.S.; OLIVEIRA, M.G.; CARLSON, R.L.R. 1998. Mathematical correlations between transverse linear skeletal dimensions obtained from computerised Ricketts cephalometric analysis. **Rev. Odonto Ciência,** 13(25): 115-130.

HERMANN, J. S.; SAKAI, A. P.C.; FRUTUOSO, J. R. C.; FRASCINO, S. V. M.; HITOS, S. F.; JÚNIOR, M. C.; AKAISHI, N. M. M.; PIGNATARI, S. S. **N. Clinical characteristics of mouth-breathing children.** Modern

Paediatrics. Sep/2013. V.49, N.9; PP:385-392.

HIGASHI, T.; SHIBA, J. K. C.; IKUTA, H. 1999. **Atlas of Oral Diagnostic Imaging.** Santos Publishing House. São Paulo, p. 56-57.

HUNGRIA, H. 1995. Nasosinusal allergic manifestations; vasomotor rhinitis; allergic rhinopathy. Chap. 9:69-78 In **Otorhinolaryngology.** 7ª ed. Ed. Guanabara-Koogan. Rio de Janeiro.

HUPP, J.R.; WILLIAMS, T. P.; VALLERAND.W. P. 1997. **Dentistry: Quick Reference.** Ed. Artes Médicas. Porto Alegre, p.490-491.

HURTADO, I. & PARINI, M. 1987. House dust mites in Caracas, Venezuela. **Ann. Allergy,** 59:128-130.

INODON, LABORATORY. 1988. **Practical manual on salivary tests for identifying people at high risk of dental caries.** Inodon Indúst. Bras. Porto Alegre, RS.

JABUR, L.B. 1998. Speech and hearing assessment. Chap. 14:283-308 In **Orthodontics. Diagnosis and Clinical Planning.(FERREIRA, F.V.** org.). 2ª ed. Artes Médicas Publishing House. São Paulo.

JULGE, K.; MUNIR, A.K.M.; VASAR, M.; BJÕRKSTÉN, B. 1998. Indoor allergen leveis and other environmental risk factors for sensitisation in Estonian homes. **Allergy,** 53:388-393.

KOGA, C.Y.; UNTERKIRCHER, C.S.; FANTINATO,V.; WATANABE, H.; JORGE, A.O.C. 1996. Influence of mouth-breather syndrome on the presence of *mutans streptococci* and *anti-streptococcus mutans* immunoglobulins in saliva. **Rev. Odontol. UNESP.,** 25(2):207-216.

KONISHI, E. & UEHARA, K. 1994. Antigen Levels of *Dermatophagoides* mites (Acari: Pyroglyphidae) in dust samples collected in homes of allergic patients. **J. Medic. Entomol.,** 31(3): 394-399.

KOVALHUK, L.C.; ROSÁRIO FILHO, N.A.; 1999. Household allergens and environmental hygiene. **Cad. Alerg. Asma Imunol., 11** (1):3-6.

LUSVARGHI, L. 1999. Identifying the mouth breather. **Rev. Assoe. Paul. Cirurg. Dent.,** 53(4):265-274.

LUZ, M.A.A.C. & BIRMAN, E.G. 1996. Caries in patients with hyposalivation: clinical, therapeutic and preventive aspects. **Rev. Bras. OdontoL, 53(6):** 27-31.

MALE, D. 1999. **Immunology - an illustrated summary.** 3ª ed. Manole. São Paulo. 129p.

MALHEIROS, M.T.S.R.; BARROS, M.A.M.T.; MACHADO, L.; AKAGAWA, Y.T.; LEÃO, R.C. 1990. Storage mites: importance in sensitising patients with respiratory allergy symptoms. **Rev. Bras. Alerg. ImunopatoL,** 13(6):233-252.

MARCHESAN, I. Q. 1998. **Fundamentals of Speech and Hearing Therapy. Clinical Aspects of Oral Motricity.** Guanabara-Koogan Publishing House. Rio de Janeiro, p. 24-35.

MARONE, S.A.M. 1997. Otorhinolaryngological Infections. Chap. 142:1658-1702. In Tratado de infectologia - Vol 2 (VERONESI, R. & FOCACCIA, R.

org.). Ed. Atheneu. São Paulo.

MAUNSELL K.; WRAITH, D.G.; CUNNINGTON, A.M. 1968. Mites and house dust allergy in bronchial asthma. **Lancei,** 15:1267-1270.

McWILL (Ed.). 1999. Allergy and the Laboratory Investigation of Allergic Processes. **Laes&Haes, 20(**116): 144-150.

MEDEIROS Jr., M.; FIGUEIREDO, J.P. 1997. Sensitisation to aeroallergens in individuals with bronchial asthma and/or chronic rhinitis in Salvador, Bahia. **Rev. Bras. Allerg. Imunopatol.,** 20:143-152.

MENDES, E. 1989. **Allergy in Brazil: Regional allergens and immunotherapy.** Manole, São Paulo, 221 pp.

MERCADANTE, M.M.N. 1998. Habits in Orthodontics. Chap. 13:255-278 In **Orthodontics. Diagnosis and Clinical Planning.(FERREIRA, F.V.** org.). 2ª ed. Artes Médicas Publishing House. São Paulo.

MILANEZI, L.A.; NAGATA, M. J. H.; FARINELLI, E. C.; STRABELLI.D. B. 1993. Mouth breathing and its periodontal implications. **Odontol. Mod.,** 20(5):25-26.

MOCELLIN, M. 1994. Mouth breathers. Chap. 8. p. 129-143. in: **Orthodontics for Speech and Hearing Therapy** (Petrelli.E.) Lovise

MORENO, L. ; CARABALLO, L. ; PUERTA, L. 1995. Medical importance of house dust mite allergens. **Biomédica,** 15:93-103.

MUMCUOGLU, Y. 1976. House dust mites in Switzerland. **J. Med. Entomol.,**

13:361-373.

MURRAY, A.B.; FERGUSON, A.C.; MORRISON, B.J. 1985. Sensitisation to house dust mites in different climatic areas. **J. Allergy Clin. Immunol.,** 76:108-112.

NASPITZ, C.; ARRUDA, L.; RIZZO, M.; BAGGIO, D.jCALDAS, E.; CHAPMAN, M.; PLATTS-MILLS, T.A.E. 1990. Mite allergy and indoor allergen exposure in asthmatic children in Brazil. **J. Allergy Clin. ImmunoL,** 85:Abs159.

NEGREIROS, B.; FILARDI,C.; TEBYRIÇÁ, J.N.; CARVALHO, L.P. 1975. House dust allergy: Comparative study with dermatophagoid extracts. **Folha Med.,** 71:385-388.

NEGREIROS, B. & ESPÍNOLA, A.B.A. 1995. Rhinitis and nasal polyposis. In NEGREIROS, B. & UNGIER, C. **Clinical Allergology.** Atheneu, São Paulo, p. 121-127.

NISHIOKA, K.; YASUEDA, H.; SAITO, H. 1998. Preventive effect of bedding encasement with microfine fibres on mite sensitisation. **J. Allergy Clin. ImmunoL, 101:** 28-32.

OLIVEIRA, C. H. ; TAKATA, L. M. H. ; JIUN, H. S. ; GRUENWALDT, J. ; GRAUDENZ, G. S. ; BARROS, P. M. G. ; PINHO Jr., J. A. ; LAZZARINI, S. 1998. Evaluation of immediate sensitivity to aeroallergens in undergraduate medical students. **Rev. Bras. Alerg. ImunopatoL, 21** (1):3- 7.

PAHO. 1989. Compendium of allergic and immunological diseases. Scientific Publication No. 513. **The Journal of the American Medical Association,** Washington, DC, USA. X+288 pp.

OSTOLAZA, M. P. 1993. **Mouth breathing in allergic rhinitis.** Monograph. National University of Rosario - Faculty of Medical Sciences - School of Speech and Hearing Therapy. 151 pp.

PARADA, R.; BAGGIO, D.; CROCE, J.; LINDIVAR, L.F. 1988. House dust mites in Santa Cruz de La Sierra, Bolivia. **Rev. Bras. Allerg. Imunopatol., 11** (5):180. Abs 123.

PASSÀLI, D. & MÕSGES, R. 1999. International Conference on Allergic Rhinitis in Childhood. **Allergy,** 54:4-34.

PEPYS, J.; CHAN, M.; HARGREAVE, F.E. 1968. Mites and house dust allergy. **Lancet,** 15:1270-1272.

PHILIP, G. & NACLERIO, R.M. 1996. Physiology and diseases of the nose. In BIERMAN, C.W. & PEARLMAN, D.S. **Allergy, Asthma and Immunology from infancy to adulthood.** 3ª ed. WB Saunders Company, Philadelphia. p. 393-410.

PLATTS-MILLS, T.A.E. & CHAPMAN, M.D. 1987. Dust mites: Immunology, allergic diseases and environmental control. **J. Allergy Clin. ImmunoL,** 80:755-775.

PLATTS-MILLS, T.A.E.; THOMAS, W.R.; AALBERSE, R.C.; VERVLOET, D.; CHAPMAN, M.D. 1992. Dust mite allergens and asthma: report of a second International workshop. **J. Allergy Clin. ImmunoL,** 89:1046-1060.

PROFFIT,W. R. 1995. Concepts of growth and development - Chap.2:18-50; The early stages of development - Chap.3:52-78; The late stages of development - Chap. 4:79-94; The aetiology of orthodontic problems - Chap.

5:95-122; Orthodontic diagnosis - The development of a problem list - Chap. 6:127-168. In
Contemporary Orthodontics. 2ª ed. Editora Guanabara Koogan. Rio de Janeiro.

QUELUZ, D.P. & GIMENEZ, C. M. M. 2000. The Mouth Breather Syndrome. **Rev. CRO-MG, 6** (1):4-9.

RIBEIRO, C.T.D. & IRULEGUI, I. 1991a. Resistance to parasitism. Chap. 6:72-81 In **Parasitologia** (Rey, L. org.). 2ª ed. Editora Guanabara-Koogan. Rio de Janeiro. XXVIII + 731 pp.

RIBEIRO, C.T.D. & IRULEGUI, I. 1991b. Execution mechanisms of the immunological response. Chap. 7:82-92 In **Parasitologia** (Rey, L. org.). 2ª ed. Editora Guanabara-Koogan. Rio de Janeiro. XXVIII + 731 pp.

RIOS, M. 1996. The mouth breather. **Rev. Faculd. Odontol. Buenos Aires,** 16(42):79-82.

RIZZO, M. C. 1998. The impact of the environment on the respiratory tract. J. **Ped., 74** (Suppl. 1):12-18.

SABRA, M.G.N. & MARTINS, E. R. 1997. Asthma and Allergic Rhinitis: Evaluation of sensitivity to the mites *Dermatophagoides spp* and *Blomia tropicalis.*
Cadernos de Alergia, Asma e Imunologia, 9(2):3-7.

SARINHO E.; FERNÁNDEZ-CALDAS, E.; JUST, E.; SOLÉ, D. 1996. House dust mites in the homes of asthmatic children and asthma controls.

city of Recife, Pernambuco. **Rev. Bras. Allerg. Imunopatol.,** 19:228- 230.

SHAFER, W. G. ; HINE, M. K. ; LEVY, B. M. 1979. Factors involved in dental caries. Chap. 7:319-369. In **Oral Pathology. 1ª** ed. Brazil, Editora Interamericana. Rio de Janeiro.

SHELDON, L. & SPECTOR, M.D. 1997. Overview of allergic rhinitis comorbidity associations. **J. Allergy Clin. Immunol.,** 99:5773-5780.

SILVA, D. S.; NETO, L. A. A. G. B.; BOUÇAS, M. F. 2000. Relationship between breastfeeding, mouth breathing and deleterious oral habits. Rev. **Flumin. Odontol.,** 6(14):25.

SMITH, T.F.; KELLY, L.B.; HEYMANN, P.W.; WILKINS, S.R.; PLATTS- MILLS, T.A.E. 1985. Natural exposure and serum antibodies to house dust mite of mite-allergic children with asthma in Atlanta. **J. Allergy Clin. Immunol., 76:792-788.**

SOLÉ, D. & SAKANO, E. (coord.). Brazilian Journal of Otorhinolaryngology. 75 (6) Nov/Dec 2012. p. 20 . Available at: <http://www.aborlccf.org.br/imageBank/consenso_sobre_rinite_-SP-2013-O4.PDF> Accessed on: 10/11/2018.

STENIUS, B.; CUNNINGTON, A.M. 1972. House dust mites and respiratory allergy: A qualitative survey of species occurring in Finnish house dust. **Scand. J. Resp. Dis.,** 53:338-348.

SUMMERS, F.M. & PRICE, D.W. 1970. Review of the mite family Cheyletidae. **Univ. Calif. Publ. Entomol.,** 61:1-153.

TENOVUO, J. & LAGERLÕF, F. 1995. Saliva. Chap.2:17-42 In **Clinical Cariology.** (THYLSTRUP, A. & FEJERSKOV, O. org.). 2ª ed. Brazil, Livraria

Santos. São Paulo. 421 pp.

THYLSTRUP, A. & FEJERSKOV, O. 1995. The oral environment - an introduction. Chap.1:13-16 In **Clinical Cariology.** 2ª ed. Brazil, Livraria Santos. São Paulo. 421 pp.

TSUJI, D.H. 1997. Infectious rhinitis. Chap. 142 - 142.3:1680-1681. **In Tratado de infectologia - Vol 2** (VERONESI, R. & FOCACCIA, R. org.). Ed. Atheneu. São Paulo.

VERVLOET, D.; PENAUD, A.; RAZZOUK, H.; SENFT, M.; ARNAUD, A.; BOUTIN.C.; CHARPIN, J. 1982. Altitude and house dust mites. **J. Allergy Clin. Immunol., 69:290-296.**

VION, P. E. 1994. **Cephalometric anatomy.** 1ª ed. Livraria Editora Santos. São Paulo, p. 42-43; 84-85.

WARNER, J.O. & WARNER, J.A. 1991. Airborne mite allergen. **Lancet,** 337:1038.

WARNER, A.; BOSTRÕN, S.; MUNIR, A.K.M.; MÕLLER, C.; SCHOU, C.; KJELLMAN, N.LM. 1998. Environmental assessment of *Dermatophagoides* mite-allergen leveis in Sweden should include Der m.1. **Allergy.,** 53:698-704.

WHARTON, G.W. 1976. House dust mites. **J. Med. Entomol.,** 6:577-621.

WHITE, S. C. & PHAROAH, M. J. 2000. **Oral Radiology. Principles and interpretation.** 4ª ed. Mosby, Inc. St. Louis, Missouri-USA. ch. 10. p. 194-198.

CHAPTER 9

ANNEXES

Annex 1: Authorisation for the work to be carried out from the patients and their guardians when they are minors:

UNIG

IGUAÇU UNIVERSITY

AUTHORISATION TO CARRY OUT RESEARCH

Me, ____

I hereby authorise the use of biological material or information provided by me for scientific purposes. I also authorise the performance of dermatological tests and the publication of the data obtained.

Nova Iguaçu, ______ de______ de.

patient's signature

UNIG

IGUAÇU UNIVERSITY

AUTHORISATION TO CARRY OUT RESEARCH

- underage patient -

Eu, ____,

legally responsible for, ______________________________ authorise the use, for scientific purposes, of biological material or information provided by me, as the person responsible, and by the patient under my legal responsibility. I also authorise dermatological tests to be carried out on the patient under my legal supervision, as well as the publication of the data obtained.

Nova Iguaçu, ____________e ____________ de____________.

____

legal representative

____

minor patient

Appendix 2: Model of the questionnaire applied to all patients:

Identification form and questionnaire:

I) Identification:

Name:

Nationality: Place of Birth:

Race: Sex: Age:

Date of birth: Telephone:

Full address:

II) Questionnaire:

1) Do you snore while you sleep? Drool on your pillow ?
2) Do you eat with your mouth open? Yes No
3) Do you breathe while chewing? Yes No
4) Do you normally have dry mouth? Yes No
5) Do you have any allergies? Yes No If yes, to what?______________

- for how long? ____

6) Do you take any medication? Yes . No Which?
7) Do you work in an air-conditioned environment? Yes No
8) Are you a restless sleeper? Yes No

9)	Do you have difficulty concentrating? Yes No
10)	Breathing: through the Mouth ? ; through the Nose ?
ADDITIONAL COMMENTS:	

Annex 3: Radiographic Examination Request: - X-rays: P.A. and Profile (requests and comparative table)

UNIG

IGUAÇU UNIVERSITY

REQUESTS FOR COMPLEMENTARY TESTS
FOR THE FINAL THESIS IN THE
MASTER'S PROGRAMME IN BIOLOGICAL SCIENCES
- PARASITIC DISEASES -

Advisor: Dr Gilberto Salles de Gazêta

Researcher: Enio Figueira Júnior

Patient:.

NECESSARY EXAMINATION(S):

1)____

2) ____

3) ____

Nova Iguaçu, _________ de_________ de_________.

____

signature of research professor

Appendix 4: Authorisation to use images

UNIG

IGUAÇU UNIVERSITY

TERM OF AUTHORISATION FOR THE USE OF IMAGES FOR RESEARCH PURPOSES

I, [patient's name], authorise the use of my image as a research participant in the research project entitled "Correlation between Mouth Breathers and Individuals with Respiratory Hypersensitivity caused by Mites", under the responsibility of Enio Figueira Júnior, linked to the Strictu-sensu Postgraduate Programme in Biological Sciences - Parasitic Diseases at Iguaçu University.

My image may only be used for analysis by the research team, presentations at professional and/or academic conferences, educational activities and the consequent scientific publications.

I am aware that there will be no dissemination of my image by any means of communication, be they television, radio or internet, except in activities linked to the teaching and research explained above. I am also aware that the researcher in charge is responsible for the safekeeping and other security procedures regarding the images.

I hereby declare that I freely and spontaneously authorise the use of my image for research purposes under the terms described above.

This document has been drawn up in two copies, one of which will be kept by the researcher and the other by you.

______________________________ ______________________________

Signature of participant | Researcher's name and signature

Nova Iguaçu, __ from ________ .

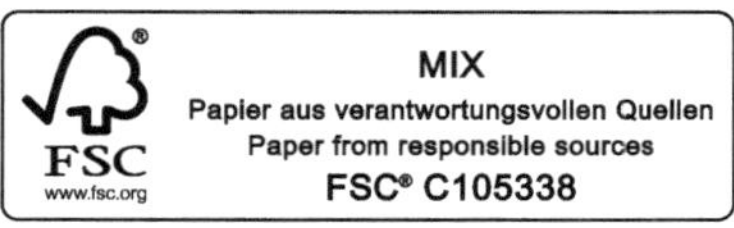

Printed by Books on Demand GmbH, Norderstedt / Germany